Workbook for Mosby's Textbook for Medication Assistants

DIANN MUZYKA PhD, RN
Clinical Associate Professor
Arizona State University
College of Nursing & Healthcare Innovation
Phoenix, Arizona

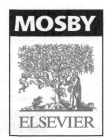

MOSBY

ELSEVIER

11830 Westline Industrial Drive
St. Louis, Missouri 63146

WORKBOOK FOR MOSBY'S TEXTBOOK FOR
MEDICATION ASSISTANTS

ISBN 978-0-323-04900-9

International Standard Book Number (ISBN) 978-0-323-04900-9

Executive Editor: Susan R. Epstein
Senior Developmental Editor: Maria Broeker
Publishing Services Manager: John Rogers
Project Manager: Cindy Thoms
Cover Designer: Jessica Williams

Working together to grow libraries in developing countries

www.elsevier.com | www.bookaid.org | www.sabre.org

ELSEVIER   BOOK AID International   Sabre Foundation

Printed in the United States of America

Last digit is the print number: 9 8 7 6 5 4 3 2 1

To my family and friends
for their encouragement and support.

Reviewers

Linda Castaldi, MNSc, RN

Division Chair
National Park Community College
Hot Springs, Arkansas

Ruth Ann Eckenstein, Med, RN

Program Specialist
Oklahoma Department of Career and Technology
    Education
Stillwater, Oklahoma

Stephen M. Setter, PharmD, CDE, CGP, FASCP

Associate Professor of Pharmocotherapy
Washington State University
Elder Services/Visiting Nurses Association
Spokane, Washington

Preface

This workbook is written to be used with *Mosby's Textbook for Medication Assistants, first edition*. It is designed to help you apply and learn the information presented in each chapter of the textbook.

Various sections are found in every chapter – **Key Terms, Circle the Best Answer, Fill in the Blanks, Matching, True/False,** and **Independent Learning Activities**. The **Key Terms** will help you identify the definitions of the key terms listed in the textbook. The **Circle the Best Answer, Fill in the Blanks, Matching,** and **True/False** sections will provide a way for you to recall the information in the textbook. Multiple-choice questions in the **Circle the Best Answer** section will, also, give you practice for taking the medication

assistant test. **Independent Learning Activities** provide practical application exercises for you to do alone or with classmates. Your instructor can give you the answers for the workbook questions. The answer key can be found in the *Instructor Resource Manual*.

Procedure Checklists that correspond with the procedures in the textbook are provided. They are intended to help you learn the procedures needed for giving medications safely.

Medication assistants-certified are important members of the health care team. Completing the exercises in this workbook will increase your knowledge, skills, and confidence. The goal is to prepare you to assist the nurse in the safe administration of drugs.

Contents

1 The Medication Assistant

Fill in the Blanks: Key Terms
Use these terms to complete questions 1–12.

Boundary crossing   Medication   Nurse practice act
Boundary signs   Medicine   Professional boundaries
Boundary violation   Medication assistant-certified (MA-C)   Professional sexual misconduct
Drug   Nursing assistive personnel   Standard of care

1. A chemical substance that has an effect on a living organism is called a _____.

2. _____ are individuals employed to give direct hands-on care and perform delegated nursing care tasks under the supervision of a licensed nurse.

3. The skills, care, and judgment required by nursing assistive personnel under similar conditions are called _____.

4. An act or behavior that meets your needs, not the person's, is called a _____.

5. Nursing assistive personnel who are allowed by state law to give drugs are called _____.

6. _____ is an act, behavior, or comment that is sexual in nature and occurs within the scope of employment.

7. Acts, behaviors, or thoughts that warn of a boundary crossing or violation are called _____.

8. Medication may also be called _____.

9. Something that separates helpful behaviors from behaviors that are not helpful is called _____.

10. A drug used to prevent and treat disease is called a _____.

11. The _____ is the law that regulates nursing practice in a state.

12. _____ is a brief act or behavior outside of the helpful zone.

Circle the BEST Answer
13. The purpose of a nurse practice act is to
    A. protect the public's welfare and safety
    B. protect the welfare of nursing assistive personnel
    C. protect health care workers
    D. protect the safety of nursing assistive personnel
14. Nursing assistive personnel
    A. may not have their certification or license revoked or suspended
    B. may practice nursing
    C. work within the legal limits of their role
    D. provide unsafe care

15. The regulatory agency responsible for nursing assistive personnel
    A. makes sure the nursing assistive personnel are incompetent
    B. makes sure that standards of care are met
    C. prevents disciplinary action if nursing assistive personnel violate a law
    D. approves all individuals as nursing assistive personnel
16. To be a medication assistant, you need the following qualifications *except*
    A. be a CNA
    B. classroom learning and clinical experiences
    C. meet program entrance requirements
    D. poor English skills
17. As an MA-C, you
    A. renew your certification as required by state law
    B. attend continuing education classes every 10 years
    C. fail to report felony convictions
    D. forget to work during your renewal period
18. As an MA-C, you
    A. follow your job description
    B. act outside the legal limits of your role
    C. give drugs by a route you did not learn
    D. only answer questions during your job interview
19. As an MA-C, you do the following *except*
    A. give drugs under the supervision of a nurse
    B. use the MAR to give and record drugs
    C. report drug side effects and adverse reactions to the nurse
    D. ignore drug errors

Fill in the Blanks
For questions 20-33 write out the meaning of each abbreviation.

20. NCSBN _____

    _____

21. RNA _____

    _____

22. EMT _____

    _____

23. LNA _____

    _____

24. MAR _____

_____

25. PRN, prn _____

_____

26. GED _____

_____

27. LPN _____

_____

28. RN _____

_____

29. IV _____

_____

30. MA-C _____

_____

31. IM _____

_____

32. LVN _____

_____

33. CNA _____

_____

34. As an MA-C, you must be able to function with reasonable skill and _____.

35. As an MA-C, you _____ and demonstrate required skills.

36. State _____ and rules limit your functions as a MA-C.

Matching
Match the type of professional boundary behavior with the correct example.

37. _____ You have sex with a patient.

38. _____ You tell a patient about your personal problems.

39. _____ You hug a person because it makes you feel good.

40. _____ You accept a gift from a patient.

A. Boundary violation
B. Professional sexual misconduct
C. Boundary crossing
D. Boundary signs

True/False
Circle T if the statement is true. Circle F if the statement is false.

41. T F   Before you work as an MA-C, you must pass a written test and skills test.

42. T F   MA-Cs can work in any health agency.

43. T F   You may refuse to follow a nurse's order if you are asked to do something beyond the legal limits of your role.

44. T F   As an MA-C, you should assist with patient care.

45. T F   An agency can limit what you can do as an MA-C.

46. T F   You may give the first dose of a newly ordered drug.

47. T F   You do not decide when to give a PRN (prn) drug.

48. T F   You decide when to hold a drug.

49. T F   You may call a doctor about a drug order.

50. T F   You may take verbal or telephone orders from a doctor.

51. T F   You may give an IV or IM drug.

Independent Learning Activities
Gather the following information about MA-Cs.
- Identify health care agencies that hire MA-Cs in your city.
  - Review job descriptions.
- List your moral or religious reasons for not giving certain drugs.
  - How would you feel about giving one of these drugs?
  - What would you say to an employer or co-worker about this?
- A nurse asks you to do something outside your scope of practice. Practice what you will say to him or her.
- You see a co-worker accept a gift. Practice what you will do in this situation.

2 Delegation

Fill in the Blanks: Key Terms
Use these terms to complete questions 1–3.

Accountable   Delegate   Nursing task

1. To _____ is to authorize another person to perform a nursing task in a certain situation.

2. Nursing care or a nursing function, procedure, activity, or work that does not require an RN's professional knowledge or judgment is called a _____

   _____.

3. Being responsible for one's actions and the actions of others who perform delegated tasks is being _____

   _____.

Circle the BEST Answer

4. When a nurse delegates a task to you, he or she must
   A. record your observations
   B. ignore your report observations
   C. tell you to ask another MA-C if you have questions about the task
   D. make sure you know how to perform the task

5. A nurse asks you to perform a task. You do the following *except*
   A. do the task even though you have not been trained
   B. restate what is expected of you
   C. contact the nurse if there is an emergency
   D. record the care given

6. Why does a nurse keep a close watch over a resident or patient?
   A. To be sure the housekeeper gave correct care
   B. To monitor the person's health status and care
   C. To make your job difficult
   D. To tell the nursing director what you did wrong

7. You should refuse to perform a task when
   A. it is within the legal limits of your role
   B. it is in your job description
   C. it is in agency policy
   D. it is a task not listed in your job description

8. Which step can the nurse delegate to you?
   A. Determining the need for PRN drugs
   B. Assessing side effects from a drug
   C. Giving certain drugs
   D. Recognizing allergic reactions

Fill in the Blanks
For questions 9-16 write out the meaning of each abbreviation.

9. CNA _____

   _____

10. LPN _____

    _____

11. LVN _____

    _____

12. MA-C _____

    _____

13. mg _____

    _____

14. NCSBN _____

    _____

15. PRN _____

    _____

16. RN _____

    _____

17. The primary role of an MA-C is to _____.

18. A nurse cannot ask you to assess a person's need for a _____.

19. You may not determine the person's need for a _____ _____ drug.

Matching
Match the example with the correct right of delegation.

20. _____ The nurse evaluates the care you give.

21. _____ The nurse delegates a task to you.

22. _____ The nurse gives you clear directions about the task.

23. _____ The nurse knows the person's physical needs when delegating to you.

24. _____ The nurse knows you have the training to perform a task safely.

A. The right task
B. The right circumstance
C. The right person
D. The right directions and communication
E. The right supervision

True/False
Circle T if the statement is true. Circle F if the statement is false.

25. T F   An RN or LPN can delegate only those tasks that are in your job description.

26. T F   The nurse who delegates a task to you is legally responsible for the task.

27. T F   As an MA-C, you can delegate a task to a CNA.

28. T F   If you perform a task that places a person at risk, you can face serious legal problems.

29. T F   A nurse needs to know your knowledge and skills before delegating a task to you.

30. T F   Feedback from the nurse is a way you can learn and improve the care you give.

Independent Learning Activities
- Obtain a copy of a job description.
  - What tasks are included in the job description?
  - What education and training are needed for the job?
- Role-play a situation in which a nurse asks you to perform a task that you should not do.

3 Ethics and Laws

Fill in the Blanks: Key Terms
Use these terms to complete questions 1–21.

Abuse
Advance directive
Assault
Battery
Civil law
Crime
Criminal law

Defamation
Ethics
False imprisonment
Fraud
Invasion of privacy
Law
Libel

Malpractice
Neglect
Negligence
Protected health information
Slander
Tort
Vulnerable adult

1. A document stating a person's wishes about health care when that person cannot make his or her own decisions is called an _____.

2. When you touch a person's body without his or her consent, it is called _____.

3. A _____ is an act that violates a criminal law.

4. Injuring a person's name and reputation by making false statements to a third person is called _____ _____.

5. Saying or doing something to trick, fool, or deceive a person is _____.

6. Making false statements in print, in writing, or through pictures or drawings is _____.

7. _____ is an unintentional wrong in which a person did not act in a reasonable and careful manner and causes harm to a person or to the person's property.

8. A _____ is a person 18 years old or older who has a disability or condition that puts him or her at risk to be wounded, attacked, or damaged.

9. The intentional mistreatment or harm of another person is _____.

10. A _____ is concerned with relationships among people.

11. Unlawful restraint or restriction of a person's freedom of movement is _____.

12. A rule of conduct made by a government body is a _____.

13. Failure to provide a person with the goods or services needed to avoid physical harm, mental anguish, or mental illness is _____.

14. A wrong committed against a person or the person's property is a _____.

15. Intentionally attempting or threatening to touch a person's body without the person's consent is _____.

16. A _____ is concerned with offenses against the public and society in general.

17. Knowledge of what is right conduct and wrong conduct is _____.

18. Violating a person's right not to have his or her name, photo, or private affairs exposed or made public without giving consent is _____.

19. Negligence by a professional person is considered _____.

20. Making false statements orally is called _____.

21. Identifying information and information about the person's healthcare that is maintained or sent in any form is _____.

Circle the BEST Answer

22. These statements are about ethics. Which is *true*?
    A. An ethical person does harm to a person.
    B. An ethical person behaves in the right way.
    C. An ethical person acts in the wrong way.
    D. An ethical person is prejudiced.

23. Which of the following is ethical behavior?
    A. Performing acts that will cause a person harm
    B. Completing each task unsafely
    C. Keeping a person's property safe
    D. Reporting errors at the end of your shift

24. The following statements are about a resident's rights. Which is *false*?
    A. Information about a drug is given in a language the person can understand.
    B. The person must take all his or her drugs.
    C. Medical and financial records are kept private.
    D. You should speak to the person in a polite manner.

25. A person has a do not resuscitate order. You do not agree with it. You
    A. ignore the person's wishes
    B. discuss the matter with the nurse
    C. ignore the doctor's order
    D. tell the person's family to have the order changed

26. Prescriptions must contain the following *except*
    A. the name and signature of the prescriber
    B. the name and address of the patient or resident
    C. the name of the insurance company
    D. the date the drug was issued
27. The following statements are about laws. Which is *false*?
    A. Civil laws are concerned with relationships among people.
    B. Criminal laws are concerned with offenses against the public.
    C. You are legally responsible for your actions.
    D. The nurse is not legally responsible for your actions.
28. Which action could lead to a charge of negligence?
    A. You gave the right drug.
    B. You gave the correct dosage of the drug.
    C. You gave the drug at the correct time.
    D. You gave the drug the wrong way.
29. To protect yourself from assault and battery, you do the following *except*
    A. explain the procedure to the person
    B. do the procedure without the person's consent
    C. stop the treatment if the person asks you to
    D. get the person's consent before doing a procedure
30. The following statements are about abuse. Which is *false*?
    A. Abuse causes physical harm.
    B. The abuser can be a spouse.
    C. Abusers are only men.
    D. Abuse can cause mental anguish.
31. Elder abuse includes the following *except*
    A. neglect
    B. involuntary seclusion
    C. financial security
    D. abandonment
32. If you suspect elder abuse, you should
    A. discuss the matter with the nurse
    B. contact the physician
    C. confront the abuser
    D. contact the social worker
33. A person burns a child on purpose. This is
    A. emotional abuse
    B. physical abuse
    C. sexual abuse
    D. substance abuse

34. A wife does not let her husband visit with family and friends. This is what type of domestic abuse?
    A. Physical
    B. Social
    C. Economic
    D. Verbal

Fill in the Blanks
For questions 35-41 write out the meaning of each abbreviation.

35. AHA _____

_____

36. DEA _____

_____

37. DNR _____

_____

38. FDA _____

_____

39. HIPAA _____

_____

40. MA-C _____

_____

41. OBRA _____

_____

42. A resident has the right to _____ and confidentiality.

43. A _____ is a document about measures that support or maintain life when death is likely.

44. _____ torts include negligence and malpractice.

45. Defamation is an example of an _____ tort.

Matching

Match the definition with the correct tort.

46. _____ A nurse gives the wrong dosage of a drug to a person.

47. _____ You give a drug to the wrong person.

48. _____ You restrain a person unlawfully.

49. _____ You make a false statement about a person in writing.

50. _____ You make a false statement about a person orally.

51. _____ You put a person's photo in the newsletter without the person's consent.

52. _____ You trick a person into taking a drug.

53. _____ You touch a person's body without the person's consent.

54. _____ You threaten to touch a person's body without the person's consent.

55. _____ You intentionally mistreat another person.

A. Slander
B. Abuse
C. Malpractice
D. Invasion of privacy
E. Assault
F. Negligence
G. Libel
H. Battery
I. Fraud
J. False imprisonment

True/False

Circle T if the statement is true. Circle F if the statement is false.

56. T   F   You should judge a person by your values.

57. T   F   You should avoid persons whose values are different from your own.

58. T   F   The FDA determines the safety of drugs before marketing.

59. T   F   The FDA ensures that manufacturers meet labeling requirements.

60. T   F   The FDA ensures that advertising standards are met when drugs are marketed.

61. T   F   The Controlled Substance Act has five classifications, or schedules, of controlled substances.

62. T   F   HIPAA protects the privacy of a person's health information.

63. T   F   Possession of a controlled substance outside of work is legal.

64. T   F   Failing to comply with the Controlled Substance Act can result in a fine or prison term.

65. T   F   If you suspect child abuse, you should share your concerns with the nurse.

Independent Learning Activities

- Write how you feel about do not resuscitate orders.
  - Does a DNR go against your personal, religious, and cultural values?
  - How will you deal with a DNR situation at work?
- Determine whether your state and agency permit MA-Cs to give schedule II drugs.
- Role-play a situation in which you observe nursing assistive personnel being disrespectful to each other.
  - How did you feel?
  - What did you do?

4 Assisting with the Nursing Process

Fill in the Blanks: Key Terms

Use these terms to complete questions 1–14.

Assessment
Evaluation
Implementation
Nursing care plan
Nursing diagnosis

Nursing intervention
Nursing process
Objective data
Observation
Planning

Signs
Subjective data
Symptoms
Vital signs

1. _____ is to perform or carry out measures in the care plan; it is a step in the nursing process.

2. A _____ is an action or measure taken by the nursing team to help the person reach a goal.

3. Using the senses of sight, hearing, touch, and smell to collect information is called _____.

4. _____ are things a person tells you about that you cannot observe through your senses; these are also called symptoms.

5. _____ is collecting information about the person; a step in the nursing process.

6. A written guide about the person's care is a _____

_____.

7. _____ is the method nurses use to plan and deliver nursing care; its five steps are assessment, nursing diagnosis, planning, implementation, and evaluation.

8. Another term for objective data is _____.

9. Temperature, pulse, respirations, blood pressure, and pain are referred to as _____.

10. _____ describes a health problem that can be treated by nursing measures; it is a step in the nursing process.

11. _____ are information that can be seen, heard, felt, or smelled; these are also called signs.

12. Another term for subjective data is _____.

13. _____ is to measure if goals in the planning step were met; it is a step in the nursing process.

14. _____ occurs when priorities and goals are set; it is a step in the nursing process.

Circle the BEST Answer

15. Which of these is *not* a step in the nursing process?
    A. Assessment
    B. Subjective data
    C. Implementation
    D. Evaluation

16. The nursing process
    A. is not important
    B. is done by doctors
    C. does not help organize nursing care
    D. helps organize nursing care

17. Which statement about a drug history is *false*?
    A. Includes prescription drugs and over-the-counter drugs
    B. Includes herbal products and street drugs
    C. Includes drug allergies
    D. Is obtained by MA-Cs

18. Which of the following is *not* objective data?
    A. A person's pulse rate
    B. The amount of urine a person voided
    C. Pain felt by a person
    D. A person's blood pressure

19. A person says, "Whenever I take this drug, I feel dizzy." This is an example of
    A. subjective data
    B. objective data
    C. a sign
    D. nursing process

20. Which observation does *not* need to be reported to the nurse at once?
    A. A change in the person's ability to respond
    B. Complaints of sudden, severe pain
    C. Vomiting
    D. Clear speech

21. The following statements are about nursing diagnosis. Which is *false*?
    A. A nursing diagnosis can relate to the side effects of a drug.
    B. A nursing diagnosis is the same as a medical diagnosis.
    C. A person can have many nursing diagnoses.
    D. A nursing diagnosis can relate to the desired effects of drugs.

22. The following statements are about planning nursing care. Which statement is *false*?
    A. The person and health team help the RN plan care.
    B. Planning involves setting priorities and goals.
    C. Planning involves setting goals.
    D. The family does not help the RN plan care.

23. Which statement about nursing interventions is *false*?
    A. Nursing interventions are chosen before goals are set.
    B. Nursing action is another term for nursing intervention.
    C. A nursing intervention does not need a doctor's order.
    D. Nursing interventions help the person reach a goal.
24. The following statements are about the care a person receives. Which statement is *false*?
    A. Care is given in the implementation step of the nursing process.
    B. You report the care given to the nurse.
    C. You record the care given in the person's medical record.
    D. Recording is done before the care is provided.
25. Which statement about vital signs is *false*?
    A. Vital signs can be affected by activity and drugs.
    B. Vital signs are measured to detect changes in normal body function.
    C. Vital signs above the normal range can be reported at the end of the shift.
    D. Vital signs below the normal range are reported to the nurse at once.
26. Which statement about taking a temperature is *false*?
    A. An oral temperature is taken if the person has diarrhea.
    B. A rectal temperature is taken if the person is unconscious.
    C. A tympanic membrane thermometer can be used if the person has ear drainage.
    D. Axillary sites are used when other sites cannot be used.
27. When taking an oral temperature, you do the following *except*
    A. permit the person to eat and smoke 15 minutes before the procedure
    B. practice hand hygiene before the procedure
    C. ask the person not to talk while taking the temperature
    D. practice hand hygiene after the procedure
28. When taking a rectal temperature, you do the following *except*
    A. lubricate the bulb end of the thermometer
    B. hold the thermometer in place as required by agency policy
    C. put on gloves
    D. force the thermometer into the rectum
29. Which statement about pulse rate is *false*?
    A. The pulse rate varies for different age groups.
    B. The normal adult pulse rate is between 60 and 100 beats per minute.
    C. A pulse rate of 56 is reported to the nurse at once.
    D. Bradycardia is a rapid pulse rate.
30. Which statement about respirations is *false*?
    A. Each respiration involves one inhalation and one exhalation.
    B. If respirations are irregular, count the rate for 30 seconds and multiply by 2.
    C. Count respirations right after taking a pulse.
    D. The healthy adult has 12 to 20 respirations a minute.

31. Which statement about blood pressures is *false*?
    A. The normal systolic pressure is less than 120 mm Hg.
    B. The normal diastolic pressure is less than 80 mm Hg.
    C. The correct size cuff is used to measure blood pressure.
    D. You may take a blood pressure on an arm with an IV or dialysis access site.
32. When measuring a person's weight, you do the following *except*
    A. weigh the person at the same time of day
    B. balance the scale at zero before weighing the person
    C. ask the person to void after being weighed
    D. ask the person to remove footwear
33. Before doing blood glucose testing, you do the following *except*
    A. be sure the procedure is in your job description
    B. obtain the necessary training
    C. guess at how to use the equipment
    D. review the procedure with the nurse
34. When measuring blood glucose, you do the following *except*
    A. check the expiration date on the reagent strip
    B. let the finger site dry after cleaning it with an anti-septic wipe
    C. discard the used lancet into the sharps container
    D. use the center, fleshy part of the fingertip for obtaining the specimen
35. For good communication, you do the following *except*
    A. use familiar words
    B. be wordy and add unnecessary information
    C. give information in a logical manner
    D. give facts and be specific
36. When recording in the medical record, you do the following *except*
    A. use ink
    B. make sure the writing is readable
    C. use correction fluid or erase when you make a mistake
    D. record only what you did and observed
37. International time is used in your agency. 1700 is what time?
    A. 7 AM
    B. 5 AM
    C. 5 PM
    D. 7 PM

Fill in the Blanks
For questions 38-47 write out the meaning of each abbreviation.

38. C _____

39. F _____

40. Hg _____

41. IV _____

_____

42. MDS _____

_____

43. mm _____

_____

44. mmHg _____

_____

45. NANDA-I _____

_____

46. OBRA _____

_____

47. OSHA _____

_____

48. Observation is using the senses of _____, _____
 _____, _____, and _____ to
 collect information.

49. The period of heart muscle contraction is called

_____.

50. The period of heart muscle relaxation is called

_____.

51. In systole, the heart is

_____.

52. In diastole, the heart is

_____.

Matching
Match the statements with the correct temperature range.

53. _____ The normal range for an oral temperature

54. _____ The normal range for a rectal temperature

55. _____ The normal range for a tympanic temperature

56. _____ The normal range for an axillary temperature

57. _____ The normal range for a temperal temperature

A. 98.6° F to 100.6° F
B. 96.6° F to 98.6° F
C. 98.6° F
D. 97.6° F to 99.6° F
E. 99.6° F

True/False
Circle T if the statement is true. Circle F if the statement is false.

58. T F   MA-Cs assist the nurse with assessment by reporting and recording what is observed about the person.

59. T F   The evaluation step of the nursing process involves measuring if the goals in the planning step were met.

60. T F   If a pulse rate is irregular, you count it for 1 minute.

61. T F   Count an apical pulse for 1 minute.

62. T F   When using a glucometer to measure blood glucose, you should follow the manufacturer's instructions.

Independent Learning Activities
• Ask to look at a nursing care plan used in your agency.
  • How often are the plans reviewed and updated?
  • Are the plans used by MA-Cs? How?
  • Do MA-Cs help develop and revise the plans? How?
• Practice taking vital signs on your classmates. Record your findings.
• Practice making observations on your classmates.
  • What did you observe about their speech?
  • What did you observe about their movement?
  • Ask them questions about the pain they have.
  • What observations can you make about their skin?
  • What observations can you make about their appetite?

5 Body Structure and Function

Fill in the Blanks: Key Terms
Use these terms to complete questions 1–15.

Artery	Hemoglobin	Metabolism	System
Capillary	Hormone	Organ	Tissue
Cell	Immunity	Peristalsis	Vein
Digestion	Menstruation	Respiration	

1. The process of supplying the cells with oxygen and removing carbon dioxide from them is called

    _____.

2. _____ is the burning of food for heat and energy by the cells.

3. A chemical substance secreted by the endocrine glands into the bloodstream is a _____.

4. The basic unit of body structure is a _____.

5. A blood vessel that carries blood away from the heart is an _____.

6. A _____ is a blood vessel that returns blood back to the heart.

7. Involuntary muscle contractions in the digestive system that move food down the esophagus through the alimentary canal is called _____.

8. _____ is the process in which the lining of the uterus breaks up and is discharged from the body through the vagina.

9. The substance in red blood cells that carries oxygen and gives blood its color is _____.

10. A _____ is a tiny blood vessel; food, oxygen, and other substances pass from the capillaries to the cells.

11. A group of cells with similar functions is

    _____.

12. Groups of tissues with the same function form a

    _____.

13. _____ is protection against a disease or condition; the person will not get or be affected by the disease.

14. The process of physically and chemically breaking down food so that it can be absorbed for use by the cells is _____.

15. Organs that work together to perform special functions form a _____.

Circle the BEST Answer

16. The following statements are about cells. Which is *false*?
    A. Cells have the same basic structure.
    B. You can see cells without a microscope.
    C. Cells need food, water, and oxygen to live.
    D. Cells are the body's building blocks.

17. The nucleus
    A. directs the cell's activities
    B. is in the center of the cell
    C. controls cell reproduction
    D. is also called a hormone

18. The following statements are about protoplasm. Which is *false*?
    A. It means "living substance."
    B. It is a semi-liquid substance much like an egg white.
    C. It refers to all structures, substances, and water within the cell.
    D. It refers to only the water within the cell.

19. The following statements are about chromosomes. Which is *false*?
    A. They are thread-like structures in the nucleus.
    B. Each cell has 23 chromosomes.
    C. Each cell has 46 chromosomes.
    D. Chromosomes contain genes.

20. The integumentary system
    A. is the largest body system
    B. has epithelial, connective, and nerve tissue
    C. is the smallest body system
    D. has oil glands and sweat glands

21. The following statements are about the epidermis. Which is *false*?
    A. It has living and dead cells.
    B. It has many blood vessels.
    C. It has few nerve endings.
    D. The living cells of the epidermis contain pigment.

22. The following statements are about the dermis. Which is *false*?
    A. It is made up of connective tissue.
    B. Blood vessels and nerves are found in the dermis.
    C. Sweat glands and oil glands are found in the dermis.
    D. Hair roots are not found in the dermis.

23. Which statement is *not* a function of the skin?
    A. It permits microorganisms and other substances to enter the body.
    B. It prevents excess amounts of water from leaving the body.
    C. It protects organs from injury.
    D. It helps regulate body temperature.
24. The musculoskeletal system
    A. provides the framework for the body
    B. lets the body move
    C. protects and gives the body shape
    D. prevents the body from moving
25. These statements are about voluntary muscles. Which is *false*?
    A. They can be consciously controlled.
    B. They are attached to bones.
    C. Arm muscles are voluntary muscles.
    D. Leg muscles are not voluntary muscles.
26. These statements are about involuntary muscles. Which is *false*?
    A. These muscles work automatically.
    B. They control the action of the stomach and intestines.
    C. They are called rough muscles.
    D. The cardiac muscle is an involuntary muscle.
27. Which statement about cerebrospinal fluid is *false*?
    A. It circulates around the brain and spinal cord.
    B. It protects the central nervous system.
    C. It lubricates movement.
    D. It cushions shocks that could easily injure brain and spinal cord structures.
28. Which statement about cranial nerves is *false*?
    A. They conduct impulses between the brain and the head, neck, chest, and abdomen.
    B. They conduct impulses for smell, vision, and hearing.
    C. They conduct impulses for pain, touch, temperature, and pressure.
    D. They conduct impulses between the brain and lower extremities.
29. The white of the eye is called the
    A. retina
    B. sclera
    C. pupil
    D. iris
30. Which statement about the ear is *false*?
    A. It is a sense organ.
    B. It secretes a waxy substance called mucus.
    C. The external ear is called the pinna or auricle.
    D. Its function is both hearing and balance.
31. The following statements are about the circulatory system. Which is *false*?
    A. It is made up of the blood, heart, and blood vessels.
    B. It carries food, oxygen, and other substances to the cells.
    C. It carries waste products to the cells.
    D. It produces and carries cells that defend the body from microbes that cause disease.

32. Which statement about the mitral valve is *true*?
    A. It is between the right atrium and the right ventricle.
    B. It allows blood flow into the atria.
    C. It is also called the tricuspid valve.
    D. It is between the left atrium and left ventricle.
33. Which statement about arteries is *false*?
    A. Arteries carry blood away from the heart.
    B. Arterial blood is rich in carbon dioxide.
    C. The aorta is the largest artery.
    D. The smallest branch of an artery is an arteriole.
34. Which statement about veins is *false*?
    A. Veins return blood to the heart.
    B. The two main veins are the inferior vena cava and the superior vena cava.
    C. Venous blood is dark red.
    D. Venous blood is rich in oxygen.
35. The lungs are protected by all the following *except*
    A. ribs
    B. sternum
    C. vertebrae
    D. epiglottis
36. In the lungs, oxygen and carbon dioxide are exchanged
    A. between the alveoli and capillaries
    B. in the bronchioles
    C. in the epiglottis
    D. between the right bronchus and the left bronchus
37. Which statement about the digestive system is *false*?
    A. It breaks down food so it can be absorbed for use by the cells.
    B. It is also called the gastro-intestinal system (GI system).
    C. It removes solid wastes from the body.
    D. It extends from the mouth to the stomach.
38. Which statement about the urinary system is *false*?
    A. It removes waste products from the blood.
    B. It maintains water balance within the body.
    C. It rids the body of carbon dioxide.
    D. It consists of the kidneys, ureters, and bladder.
39. A person feels the need to urinate when the bladder contains about
    A. 125 ml of urine
    B. 250 ml of urine
    C. 500 ml of urine
    D. 1000 ml of urine
40. Which statement about testosterone is *false*?
    A. It is produced in the testes.
    B. It is needed for reproductive organ function.
    C. It is needed for the development of the male secondary sex characteristics.
    D. It is needed for ovulation.
41. Which statement about estrogen and progesterone is *false*?
    A. They are secreted by the ovaries.
    B. They are needed for reproductive system function.
    C. They are needed for the development of female secondary sex characteristics.
    D. They are needed for ejaculation.

42. The master gland is the
   A. thyroid gland
   B. parathyroid gland
   C. pituitary gland
   D. adrenal gland
43. The thyroid hormone regulates
   A. growth
   B. metabolism
   C. calcium use
   D. fertilization
44. Which statement about insulin is *false*?
   A. It is secreted by the pancreas.
   B. It regulates the amount of sugar in the blood available for use by the cells.
   C. It is needed for sugar to enter the cells.
   D. It is secreted by the stomach.
45. The function of the immune system is to
   A. protect organs from injury
   B. regulate body temperature
   C. protect the body from disease and infection
   D. provide a framework for the body

Fill in the Blanks
For questions 46-55 write out the meaning of each abbreviation.

46. ACTH _____

47. ADH _____

48. CNS _____

49. GH _____

50. GI _____

51. mL _____

52. RBC _____

53. TH _____

54. TSH _____

55. WBC _____

56. The integumentary system is also called _____

57. The outer layer of the skin is the _____

58. The inner layer of the skin is the _____

59. When you are angry, scared, excited, or exercising, the _____ nervous system is stimulated.

60. The _____ nervous system is activated when you relax.

61. Red blood cells (RBCs) are called _____

62. White blood cells (WBCs) are called _____

63. Upon entering the lungs, the bronchi divide many times into smaller branches called _____

64. When the bronchioles subdivide, they end up in tiny one-celled air sacs called _____

Matching
Match the cell structure with the correct definition.

65. _____ The outer covering that encloses the cell and helps it hold its shape.
66. _____ The control center of the cell.
67. _____ The structure that contains smaller structures that perform cell functions.
68. _____ Structures, substances, and water within the cell.

A. Nucleus
B. Protoplasm
C. Cytoplasm
D. Cell membrane

Match the statement to the correct type of tissue.

69. _____ Tissue lining the nose, mouth, respiratory tract, stomach, and intestines.
70. _____ Tissue that anchors, connects, and supports other tissues.
71. _____ Tissue that stretches and contracts to let the body move.
72. _____ Tissue that receives and carries impulses to the brain and back to body parts.
73. _____ A thick layer of fat and connective tissue.

A. Subcutaneous
B. Muscle tissue
C. Connective tissue
D. Epithelial tissue
E. Nerve tissue

Match the statement with the correct type of bone.

74. _____ These bones bear the body's weight.

75. _____ These bones allow skill and ease in movement.

76. _____ These bones protect the organs.

77. _____ These bones allow various degrees of movement and flexibility.

A. Irregular bones
B. Long bones
C. Flat bones
D. Short bones

Match the statement with the correct term.

78. _____ The point at which two or more bones meet.

79. _____ The connective tissue at the end of the long bones.

80. _____ It lines the joints.

81. _____ Strong bands of connective tissue.

A. Synovial membrane
B. Joint
C. Cartilage
D. Ligaments

Match the statement with the type of joint.

82. _____ Allows movement in all directions.

83. _____ Allows movement in one direction.

84. _____ Allows turning from side to side.

A. Pivot joint
B. Ball-and-socket joint
C. Hinge joint

Match the statement with the correct term.

85. _____ Receives blood from body tissues.

86. _____ Receives blood from the lungs.

87. _____ Pumps blood to the lungs for oxygen.

88. _____ Pumps blood to all parts of the body.

A. Left ventricle
B. Left atrium
C. Right ventricle
D. Right atrium

True/False

Circle T if the statement is true. Circle F if the statement is false.

89. T   F   The process of cell division is called mitosis.

90. T   F   Mitosis is needed for tissue growth and repair.

91. T   F   Bones, tendons, ligaments, and cartilage are connective tissue.

92. T   F   The epidermis and dermis are supported by subcutaneous tissue.

93. T   F   Hair in the nose and ears protect these organs from dust and insects.

94. T   F   Nails protect the tips of the fingers and toes.

95. T   F   Sweat glands help the body regulate temperature.

96. T   F   The body is heated as sweat evaporates.

97. T   F   Oil glands help keep the hair and skin rough and dull.

98. T   F   Nerve endings in the skin help protect the body from injury.

99. T   F   Bones, joints, and muscles are part of the musculoskeletal system.

100. T   F   Bones are covered by a membrane called periosteum.

101. T   F   Blood cells are formed in the bone marrow.

102. T   F   The nervous system controls, directs, and coordinates body functions.

103. T   F   The central nervous system consists of the brain and spinal cord.

104. T   F   The peripheral nervous system involves the nerves throughout the body.

105. T   F   The spinal cord contains pathways that conduct messages to and from the brain.

106. T   F   Glands in the auditory canal secrete a waxy substance called cerumen.

107. T   F   Hemoglobin in red blood cells carries oxygen to the cells.

108. T   F   Leukocytes protect the body against infection.

109. T   F   Platelets (thrombocytes) carry carbon dioxide to cells.

110. T   F   The respiratory system brings carbon dioxide into the lungs and removes oxygen from the lungs.

111. T   F   The trachea is also called the windpipe.

112. T   F   The lungs are separated from the abdominal cavity by a muscle called the diaphragm.

113. T   F   Each lung is covered by a two-layered sac called the pleura.

114. T   F   Digestion begins in the stomach.

115. T   F   Peristalsis moves food down the esophagus through the alimentary canal.

116. T   F   The ureters carry urine from the kidneys to the bladder.

117. T   F   The prostate gland lies just below the bladder.

118. T   F   Calcium is needed for nerve and muscle function.

119. T   F   Insufficient amounts of calcium cause tetany.

120. T   F   The gonads are the glands of human reproduction.

Independent Learning Activities
- Using your own body, move joints of each type to see how they move.
- Listen to your chest with a stethoscope. What sounds do you hear?
- Listen to your abdomen with a stethoscope. What sounds do you hear?

6 Basic Pharmacology

Fill in the Blanks: Key Terms
Use these terms to complete questions 1–25.

Adverse drug reaction (ADR)
Allergic reaction
Anaphylactic reaction
Anaphylaxis
Desired action
Dilute
Drug blood level
Drug interaction
Drug reaction

Enteral route
Generic name
Hives
Idiosyncratic reaction
Intramuscular (IM)
Intravenous (IV)
Parenteral route
Percutaneous route
Pharmacology

Placebo
Reconstitute
Side effect
Subcutaneous
Toxicity
Trademark
Urticaria

1. An unfavorable response to a substance that causes a hyper-sensitivity reaction is an _____.

2. The _____ is the amount of a drug present in the blood.

3. Another term for urticaria is _____.

4. The _____ gives drugs through the skin or a mucous membrane.

5. _____ is the exposure to large amounts of a substance that should not cause problems in smaller amounts; the reaction when side effects are severe.

6. _____ is characterized by raised, irregularly shaped patches on the skin and severe itching; also called hives.

7. An unintended effect on the body from using a legal drug, illegal drug, or two or more drugs; this drug reaction is called an _____.

8. To _____ is to add the correct amount of water or other liquid.

9. The drug's common name is its _____.

10. _____ means *within a vein*.

11. To _____ is to add water or other liquid to a powder or solid form of a drug.

12. The _____ is the brand name or trade name of the drug.

13. An expected response is a _____.

14. A _____ may also be called an adverse drug reaction.

15. To give a drug _____ is to give it within a muscle.

16. _____ is the study of drugs and their actions on living organisms.

17. An _____ is another term for anaphylaxis.

18. When the action of one drug is altered by the action of another drug, it is a _____.

19. Something unusual or abnormal that happens when a drug is first given is an _____.

20. Drugs given by the _____ bypass the GI tract.

21. A drug dosage form that has no active ingredients is a _____.

22. A _____ is an unintended reaction to a drug given in a normal dosage.

23. The _____ gives drugs directly into the gastro-intestinal (GI) tract.

24. _____ is a severe, life-threatening sensitivity to an antigen; this is also known as an anaphylactic reaction.

25. _____ means *beneath the skin*.

Circle the BEST Answer
26. The trade name of a drug is its
    A. chemical name
    B. generic name
    C. official name
    D. brand name

27. The following statements refer to drug classifications. Which is *false*?
    A. Drugs may be classified according to the body system they affect.
    B. The physiologic action relates to what the drug does in the body.
    C. Clinical indications relate to the signs or reasons for using a drug.
    D. Illegal drugs are approved for use by the FDA.

28. Drugs that interact with a receptor to cause a response are
    A. antagonists
    B. partial agonists
    C. agonists
    D. receptors

29. Metabolism refers to the
    A. process by which a drug is transferred from its site of body entry to circulating body fluids (blood, lymph) for distribution
    B. way drugs are transported by circulating body fluids to the sites of action (receptors) and to the sites of metabolism and excretion
    C. process by which the body inactivates drugs
    D. elimination of a drug from the body
30. The rate of absorption depends on the following *except*
    A. the route of administration
    B. blood flow through the tissue where the drug was given
    C. how well the drug can dissolve (solubility)
    D. the clinical indications for using a drug
31. To promote absorption, you do the following *except*
    A. give oral drugs with minimal water
    B. give oral drugs with enough fluid
    C. reconstitute and dilute drugs as recommended by the manufacturer
    D. give drugs into the correct tissue
32. Which route is *not* an enteral route?
    A. oral
    B. skin
    C. rectal
    D. nasogastric
33. Which route is *not* a parenteral route?
    A. subcutaneous
    B. intramuscular
    C. intraocular
    D. intravenous
34. Which of the following is *not* a percutaneous route?
    A. drugs given by inhalation
    B. drugs given under the tongue
    C. drugs given into the muscle
    D. drugs given on the skin
35. If the drug blood level is low, you know the
    A. dosage will be reduced
    B. person may show signs of toxicity
    C. dosage may be increased
    D. dosage will be given less often
36. Which statement about metabolism is *false*?
    A. The liver is the primary site for drug metabolism.
    B. Illness and age may affect metabolism.
    C. The use of other drugs may affect metabolism.
    D. The stomach is the primary site for drug metabolism.
37. The primary routes for excretion of drugs are
    A. saliva and breast milk
    B. urine and feces
    C. skin and lungs
    D. mucus and tears
38. The following statements are about side effects. Which is *false*?
    A. Side effects are desired.
    B. Nausea and dry mouth are common side effects.
    C. Dizziness is a common side effect.
    D. Blurred vision and ringing in the ears are common side effects.

39. The following statements are about drug reactions. Which is *false*?
    A. Most can be prevented.
    B. They are a leading cause of death in the United States.
    C. Rash and itching are common drug reactions.
    D. Blurred vision and ringing in the ears are common drug reactions.
40. A person has an anaphylactic reaction to a drug. Which statement is *false*?
    A. It is a medical emergency.
    B. The person may use the drug again.
    C. Signs and symptoms can occur within seconds.
    D. Signs and symptoms may include sweating, dyspnea, and irregular pulse.
41. A person has a mild allergic reaction to a drug. The person does the following *except*
    A. receive information about the drug
    B. use the drug again
    C. tell health professionals about the reaction
    D. wear a medical-alert bracelet or necklace that explains the allergy
42. You are giving a drug you are not familiar with. Which resource would you *not* use?
    A. *American Hospital Formulary Service, Drug Information*
    B. *Clinical Nursing Skills*
    C. Manufacturer package inserts
    D. *Physician's Desk Reference (PDR)*

Fill in the Blanks
For questions 43-51 write out the meaning of each abbreviation.

43. ADME _____

44. ADR _____

45. CNS _____

46. GI _____

47. FDA _____

48. IM _____

49. IV _____

50. OTC _____

51. PDR _____

_____.

52. The process by which the body inactivates drugs is called _____.

53. The elimination of a drug from the body is _____

_____.

54. A drug resource must be accurate and _____

_____.

True/False
Circle T if the statement is true. Circle F if the statement is false.

55. T   F   Non-prescription drugs are also called over-the-counter (OTC) drugs.

56. T   F   Drugs change a physiologic activity within the body.

57. T   F   Usually a drug forms chemical bonds within specific sites in the body.

58. T   F   A drug must dissolve in body fluids before it can be absorbed into body tissue.

59. T   F   A blood sample may be studied to determine the amount of a drug present in the blood.

60. T   F   Drugs usually affect only one body system.

61. T   F   The most common allergic reaction to a drug is urticaria.

62. T   F   Age, body weight, and illness may affect a person's response to drugs.

63   T   F   A placebo is commonly called a "sugar pill."

64. T   F   Drug interactions are always harmful.

Independent Learning Activities
- Look at several drug bottles.
  - What drug names appear on the bottles?
  - What information is provided on the bottles?
- What drug resources are available on your nursing unit?
  - What information is in each resource?
- Ask the nurse for package inserts for drugs.
  - What does the package insert tell you about the drug?

7 Life Span Considerations

Fill in the Blanks: Key Terms
Use these terms to complete questions 1–7.

Absorption   Excretion   Therapeutic drug monitoring
Distribution   Metabolism
Enzymes   Metabolite

1. _____ are substances produced by
   body cells; using oxygen, they break down glucose
   and other nutrients to release energy for cellular work.

2. The measurement of a drug's concentration in body
   fluids is _____.

3. _____ is the process by which a
   drug is transferred from its site of body entry to
   circulating body fluids (blood, lymph) for distribution.

4. A product of drug metabolism is _____.

5. The elimination of a drug from the body is

   _____.

6. The way drugs are transported by circulating body
   fluids to the sites of action (receptors) and to the sites
   of metabolism and excretion is _____.

7. _____ is the process by which the
   body in-activates drugs.

Circle the BEST Answer

8. Absorption of topical drugs is usually effective in
   infants. Why?
   A. The skin is more fully hydrated (has more water).
   B. The skin is dryer.
   C. The skin is more wrinkled.
   D. There is a decreased number of hair follicles.

9. Which factor enhances topical drug absorption in
   older persons?
   A. Thin skin
   B. Dry skin
   C. Wrinkled skin
   D. Decreased number of hair follicles

10. A tablet is too large for a person to swallow. You
    A. crush the tablet
    B. order a liquid form of the drug
    C. ask the nurse's permission to crush the tablet
    D. do not give the drug

11. Which statement about crushing drugs is *false*?
    A. Crushing certain drugs affects the absorption rate.
    B. Timed-released tablets may be crushed.
    C. Enteric-coated tablets are not crushed.
    D. Sublingual tablets are not crushed.

12. A person has a chewable drug. You should
    A. determine if the person is asleep
    B. ask about loose teeth
    C. ask if the person has dentures
    D. ask if the person has cavaties

13. Gastro-intestinal absorption of drugs is influenced by
    all the following *except*
    A. how much acid is in the stomach
    B. how fast the stomach empties
    C. how fast digested food and fluids move through
       the GI tract
    D. how much fluid is in the stomach

14. Drug metabolism is affected by all the following
    factors *except*
    A. enzymes
    B. smoking
    C. diet
    D. exercise

15. As kidney function decreases, the doctor may
    A. order kidney function tests
    B. decrease drug dosages
    C. increase drug dosages
    D. give the drug less often

16. Which statement about therapeutic drug monitoring
    is *false*?
    A. It is done to measure a drug's concentration in
       body fluids.
    B. Blood testing is commonly used.
    C. Therapeutic drug monitoring is essential for all
       drugs.
    D. Therapeutic drug monitoring is essential for
       persons with certain health problems.

17. You assist with monitoring the effects of drug therapy
    by doing the following *except*
    A. take accurate vital signs
    B. report abnormal vital signs at once
    C. measure urinary output accurately
    D. measure gastric pH inaccurately

18. The following statements are about children on drug
    therapy. Which is *false*?
    A. Accurate height and weight measurements are
       important.
    B. Appropriate devices are used when giving liquid
       drugs.
    C. Dilute oral drugs in powder form according to the
       manufacturer's instructions.
    D. Allergic reactions occur slowly in children.

19. To assist an older person with drug therapy, you should
    A. use drug organizers and calendars to keep track of
       when to take drugs
    B. tell the person to keep all old drugs
    C. crush timed-released tablets
    D. never break a tablet in half if there is a "score"
       mark on the tablet

20. A pregnant woman should do the following *except*
    A. try non-drug treatments first
    B. take herbal medicines
    C. take only drugs ordered by the doctor
    D. avoid drinking alcohol

Fill in the Blanks

21. How much acid is in the stomach is referred to as ___

    _____ .

True/False
Circle T if the statement is true. Circle F is the statement is false.

24. T   F   Drug metabolism is faster in older adults.

25. T   F   GI motility is decreased in older persons.

26. T   F   The nurse may involve family members and caregivers when teaching a person about his or her drugs.

27. T   F   When taking drugs, breast-feeding mothers need to know about adverse effects that might occur in the infant.

28. T   F   All drugs may be crushed.

Independent Learning Activities
- Ask the nurse to show you a scored tablet, a timed-release tablet, an enteric-coated tablet, and a sublingual tablet.
- Ask the nurse to show you a medication cup, an oral dropper, and an oral syringe.
- Role-play giving a drug to an infant, a toddler, and a pre-school child.
- Ask the nurse to show you how to crush drugs according to your agency's policy.

22. How fast the stomach empties is known as _____

    _____ .

23. How fast digested food and fluids move through the GI tract is called _____

    _____ .

8 Drug Orders and Prescriptions

Fill in the Blanks: Key Terms

Use these terms to complete questions 1–10.

Chart   Medication order   Standing order
Clinical record   Prescription   STAT order
Drug order   PRN order
Medical record   Single order

1. The _____ is the written account of a person's condition and response to treatment and care; also known as the chart or clinical record.

2. A _____ permits a drug to be given for a certain number of doses or for a certain number of days.

3. A _____ is a drug order written for a person leaving the hospital or nursing center or for a person seen in a clinic or doctor's office; it is written on a prescription pad or it is called in, faxed, or e-mailed to the pharmacy by the doctor.

4. A _____ requires the drug to be given at once and only one time.

5. A _____ is another term for medical record.

6. A _____ is written on the agency's (hospital, nursing center) physician's order form for a patient or resident; it is also known as a medication order.

7. For a _____, the nurse decides when to give the drug based on the person's needs.

8. Another term for medical record is _____.

9. A _____ is used when a drug is to be given at a certain time and only one time.

10. A _____ is the same as a drug order.

Circle the BEST Answer

11. A drug is ordered STAT. You will give the drug
    A. after lunch
    B. immediately
    C. after break
    D. after talking with the doctor

12. An antibiotic is ordered daily for 10 days. The doctor must renew the order if he or she wants the drug to be given longer. This is an example of a
    A. STAT order
    B. single order
    C. standing order
    D. PRN order

13. A person has a headache and the nurse decides to give a drug. This is an example of a
    A. STAT order
    B. single order
    C. standing order
    D. PRN order

14. A doctor begins to give you a drug order. You do the following *except*
    A. politely give your name and title and ask the doctor to wait for a nurse
    B. promptly find a nurse to speak with the doctor
    C. accept the verbal order from the doctor
    D. politely tell the doctor you cannot accept the order

15. Which abbreviation is on the "Do Not Use" list?
    A. a.c.
    B. gtt
    C. h.s.
    D. t.i.d.

16. The Roman numeral X equals
    A. 1
    B. 5
    C. 10
    D. 50

17. How many teaspoons are in 1 tablespoon?
    A. 1
    B. 2
    C. 3
    D. 4

18. The following statements are about standard drug administration times. Which is *false*?
    A. They help prevent drug errors.
    B. They help make sure drugs are given safely and on time.
    C. The times are the same in all agencies.
    D. Always follow the standard times used in your agency.

19. The following statements are about prescription labels. Which is *false*?
    A. Always read the label carefully.
    B. If a label is not complete, tell the nurse at once.
    C. Check the expiration date.
    D. You may give a drug after the expiration date.

20. Which statement about a medical record is *false*?
    A. It is a legal document.
    B. Each form is stamped with the person's name and other identifying information.
    C. Agencies have policies about medical records and who can see them.
    D. You have an ethical and legal duty to share the person's information with anyone.

21. Which statement about an MAR is *false*?
    A. It lists only the oral drugs to be given to a person.
    B. It provides a space for recording the time the drug was given.
    C. It provides a space to record who gave the drug.
    D. It includes a place to note the person's allergies.
22. When do you record a drug as given on the MAR?
    A. At the end of the shift
    B. At once after giving the drug
    C. After the CNA gives the drug
    D. After all drugs are given
23. A person has an allergy to a drug listed on the MAR. You should
    A. tell the nurse at once
    B. give the drug
    C. call the doctor
    D. tell the unit secretary
24. Which statement about transcribing drug orders is *false*?
    A. Make sure your state and agency allow you to transcribe drug orders.
    B. Use only the drug times approved for use in your agency.
    C. Write clearly and neatly.
    D. Use an abbreviation from the "Do Not Use" list.

Fill in the Blanks
For questions 25-31 write out the meaning of each abbreviation.

25. ISMP _____

26. IV _____

27. MAR _____

28. PRN _____

29. STAT _____

30. TO _____

31. VO _____

Fill in the Blanks
For questions 32-39 write out the meaning of each drug administration time.

32. b.i.d. _____

33. t.i.d. _____

34. q.i.d. _____

35. q.6.h. _____

36. q.8.h. _____

37. q.12.h. _____

38. a.c. _____

39. p.c. _____

Matching
Match the type of order with the correct definition.

40. _____ The doctor writes the order on the physician's order form or prescription pad.

41. _____ The doctor gives the order orally to a nurse.

42. _____ The doctor gives the order to a nurse over the phone.

43. _____ An order is faxed from a doctor's office to the nursing unit on which the person is a patient or resident.

44. _____ The doctor enters the order into a computer.

A. Verbal order (VO)
B. Faxed order
C. Electronic order
D. Written order
E. Telephone order (TO)

True/False
Circle T if the statement is true. Circle F if the statement is false.

45. T   F   The doctor needs to sign a drug order that was faxed to your nursing unit.

46. T   F   Before giving a drug, you always read the drug label carefully.

47. T   F   You record a PRN drug right after you give it.

Independent Learning Activities
- Review the list of approved abbreviations in your agency.
- Review the list of "Do Not Use" abbreviations in your agency.
- What are the standard drug administration times in your agency?
- Review prescription labels. Did you find any with missing information?
- Review the forms in the medical record in your agency.
  - On which forms do you record information?
- Ask a nurse to allow you to observe as he or she verifies and transcribes drug orders. After observing, discuss the process with the nurse.

9 Medication Safety

Fill in the Blanks: Key Terms
Use these terms to complete questions 1–5.

Dose   Infection   Route

Drug diversion   Medication reminder

1. An _____ is a disease state resulting from the invasion and growth of microbes in the body.

2. How and where the drug enters the body is the _____ _____.

3. The amount of drug to give is the _____.

4. A _____ reminds the person to take drugs, observes them being taken as prescribed, and charts that they were taken.

5. Taking a person's drugs for your own use is _____.

Circle the BEST Answer

6. Medication safety involves all the following *except*
   A. correct dispensing of the drug
   B. making errors in drug administration
   C. correct storage of the drug
   D. correct disposal of the drug

7. When drugs are received from the pharmacy, you should do the following *except*
   A. compare the pharmacy label against the drug order on the MAR
   B. check that the number of doses is correct
   C. tell the nurse if the number of doses is not correct
   D. take the drug for your own use

8. Frequently used drugs are kept on the nursing unit in your agency. This is called
   A. floor or ward stock system
   B. unit dose system
   C. computer-controlled dispensing system
   D. individual prescription order system

9. Which statement about the computer-controlled dispensing system is *false*?
   A. A security code and password are used to access the system.
   B. The system is safe and time efficient.
   C. The system is cheap.
   D. The system uses a bar code.

10. These statements are about controlled substances. Which is *false*?
    A. Federal laws regulate their use.
    B. They are kept in a locked cabinet or in a locked drawer.
    C. An inventory control sheet is used to account for each drug and dose given.
    D. They are kept in the person's drug drawer.

11. Only a portion of a controlled substance dose is ordered. What should you do with the unused portion?
    A. Return it to the pharmacy.
    B. Return it to the medicine room.
    C. Ask a nurse to watch you dispose of the unused portion.
    D. Save the unused portion for the next dose.

12. To properly store drugs, you do all the following *except*
    A. keep drug containers closed tightly
    B. store drugs in their original containers or unit dose packets
    C. open two or more bins or drawers at a time
    D. store drugs as noted on the label or unit dose packet

13. A drug is dropped on the floor or bed. What should you do?
    A. Give it to the person.
    B. Keep it for yourself.
    C. Dispose of the drug following agency policy.
    D. Return it to the drug box.

14. The following statements are about drug disposal. Which is *false*?
    A. Follow agency policy for drug disposal.
    B. You should have someone watch you dispose of a drug.
    C. Record the name and title of the person who witnessed you dispose the drug.
    D. You should dispose of a drug by yourself.

15. When would you *not* read the drug label?
    A. Before removing the drug from the cart or shelf
    B. Before preparing or measuring the prescribed dose
    C. Before returning the drug to the shelf
    D. Before charting

16. Your agency permits drugs to be given 30 minutes before the scheduled time and 30 minutes after the scheduled time. If a drug is ordered for 0800, you can give it
    A. between 0830 and 0930
    B. between 0730 and 0830
    C. between 0845 and 0945
    D. between 0700 and 0900

17. A person has a drug ordered PRN. You do the following *except*
    A. make sure no one else gave the drug
    B. record the drug at the end of the shift on the MAR
    C. check the person's MAR and chart
    D. make sure that the right amount of time between doses has passed

18. To give the right dose, you
   A. compare the dose on the pharmacy label against the MAR
   B. compare the dose on the pharmacy label against the Kardex
   C. compare the dose on the pharmacy label against the progress notes
   D. compare the dose on the pharmacy label against the graphic sheet
19. The doctor ordered 100 mg of the drug. The drug is supplied in 50-mg tablets. How many tablets will you give?
   A. 1
   B. 2
   C. 3
   D. 4
20. To make sure you have the right person, you
   A. use at least two identifiers
   B. check only the person's name
   C. check the person's room number
   D. check the person's bed number
21. The following statements are about identifying the right person. Which is *false*?
   A. Identify the person every time you give a drug.
   B. Call the person by name when checking the ID bracelet.
   C. Identify the person right before you give the drug.
   D. Identify the person and then leave the room to get the drug or to collect supplies.
22. Which route has the most rapid onset of action?
   A. intravenous
   B. intramuscular
   C. subcutaneous
   D. oral
23. The drug on the MAR is oral. The pharmacy label is IM. What should you do?
   A. Give the drug orally.
   B. Give the drug IM.
   C. Check with the nurse.
   D. Call the doctor.
24. You are to give an oral drug to a person who is having difficulty swallowing today. What will you do?
   A. Tell the nurse.
   B. Call the doctor.
   C. Ask a family member to give the drug.
   D. Ask a friend to give the drug.
25. You can prevent drug errors by doing the following *except*
   A. never leave a drug unattended
   B. make sure you have good lighting
   C. tell other staff members it is okay to interrupt you
   D. stay with the person to make sure that all drugs have been swallowed
26. Which of the following is an example of a drug error?
   A. giving a drug at the right time
   B. giving the drug in the right way
   C. recording that a drug was given
   D. missing or skipping a dose

27. If you do make a drug error, you do the following *except*
   A. complete an incident report
   B. follow agency policy about describing what happened
   C. give your opinions or thoughts about why the error happened
   D. tell the nurse

Fill in the Blanks
For questions 28-46 write out the meaning of each abbreviation.

28. ADE ___
29. ALR ___
30. CDC ___
31. FDA ___
32. HBV ___
33. HIV ___
34. ID ___
35. IM ___
36. ISMP ___
37. IV ___
38. MAR ___
39. mg ___
40. NDC ___
41. OPIM ___
42. OSHA ___

43. PPE _____

_____

44. PRN _____

_____

45. STAT _____

_____

46. subcut _____

_____

In questions 47-52 list the Six Rights of Drug Administration.

47. Right _____
48. Right _____
49. Right _____
50. Right _____
51. Right _____
52. Right _____

True/False
Circle T if the statement is true. Circle F if the statement is false.

53. T F   The individual prescription order system is used in your agency. This means the pharmacy sends a 3- to 5-day supply of an ordered drug to the nursing unit for the person.

54. T F   The unit dose system provides a single dose of a drug in one package.

55. T F   A narcotic count is done at the end of a shift by two nurses going off-duty.

56. T F   During the narcotics count, unopened boxes and containers are inspected for tampering.

57. T F   If you leave the drug cart to enter a person's room, you should lock the cart.

58. T F   Drug cart keys may be kept on the cart when you enter a person's room.

59. T F   Drugs may be stored in a refrigerator with food or fluids.

60. T F   Narcotics are double-locked.

61. T F   You can assume that the pharmacist provided you with the right drug.

62. T F   Before giving any drug, compare the exact spelling of the drug with the MAR.

63. T F   For very simple drug calculations, you do not need to have a nurse check the dose.

64. T F   You may change the route of administration of a drug.

65. T F   You may change the dosage of a drug.

66. T F   You must record giving a drug as soon as possible.

67. T F   You record when a drug was not given and why.

68. T F   If a person refuses to take a drug, you record the reason for the refusal.

69. T F   You record a drug before it is taken by the person.

70. T F   When giving drugs, you do not need to be concerned about getting infections.

71. T F   Practice hand hygiene before and after giving drugs.

72. T F   Drug diversion is a crime.

Independent Learning Activities
- Review your state laws and your job description.
  - Are you permitted to do drug calculations?
  - By which routes may you give drugs?
  - May you give controlled substances?
- Role-play giving drugs, following the Six Rights of Drug Administration.
- Review the rules of hand hygiene in the textbook.

10 Oral, Sublingual, and Buccal Drugs

Fill in the Blanks: Key Terms
Use these terms to complete questions 1–15.

Buccal
Capsule
Elixir
Emulsion

Lavage
Lozenge
Medicine cup
Medicine dropper

Souffle cup
Sublingual
Suspension
Syringe

Syrup
Tablet
Troche

1. A small paper or plastic cup used for solid drug forms is a _____.

2. An _____ is an oral dose form containing small droplets of water-in-oil or oil-in-water.

3. A _____ drug is placed inside the cheek.

4. A liquid containing solid drug particles is a _____.

5. Washing out the stomach is called a _____.

6. An oral dose form containing a drug dissolved in sugar is a _____.

7. A _____ is a flat disk containing a medicinal agent with a flavored base.

8. A gelatin container that holds a drug in a dry powder or liquid is a _____.

9. A _____ is a plastic measuring device with three parts—tip, barrel, and plunger.

10. A small glass or plastic tube with a hollow rubber ball at one end is a _____.

11. An _____ is a clear liquid made up of a drug dissolved in alcohol and water.

12. A _____ drug is placed under the tongue.

13. A plastic container with measurement scales is a _____ _____.

14. Another term for lozenge is _____.

15. A dried, powdered drug compressed into a small disk is a _____.

Circle the BEST Answer
16. The following statements are about oral drugs. Which is *false*?
    A. They are easy to give.
    B. They have the longest rate of absorption.
    C. They have the slowest onset of action.
    D. Some can harm or discolor teeth.
17. Which person would you give an oral drug to?
    A. The person who is unconscious
    B. The person who is conscious
    C. The person who is vomiting
    D. The person with gastric suction

18. Which of the following drug orders would you question?
    A. 50 mg PO
    B. 50 mg orally
    C. 50 mg by mouth
    D. 50 mg per os
19. A person is receiving a timed-release capsule. This means
    A. more doses are needed per day
    B. all the granules inside the capsule dissolve at the same time
    C. there is a continuous release of the drug
    D. it is the same as any other capsule
20. Enteric-coated tablets dissolve in the
    A. stomach
    B. mouth
    C. small intestine
    D. rectum
21. Which dose form is *not* a liquid?
    A. Elixir
    B. Emulsion
    C. Syrup
    D. Troche
22. When giving a drug with a medicine dropper, you should
    A. turn the dropper upside down
    B. only use the dropper supplied by the manufacturer of the drug
    C. transfer the drug from the medicine dropper to another container
    D. use any dropper you can find
23. A person is to receive 1 tablespoon of a drug. You will give
    A. 10 mL
    B. 15 mL
    C. 20 mL
    D. 25 mL
24. A person is to receive 1 teaspoon of a drug. You will give
    A. 1 mL
    B. 2 mL
    C. 4 mL
    D. 5 mL
25. A person is to receive 1 ounce of a drug. You will give
    A. 10 mL
    B. 15 mL
    C. 30 mL
    D. 35 mL

26. When giving oral drugs, you do the following *except*
    A. give solid drugs before liquid drugs
    B. mix solid drugs with liquid drugs
    C. stay with the person while he or she takes the drug
    D. place a bottle lid upside down on a clean surface
27. Which of the following drugs will you give first?
    A. The liquid drug
    B. The lozenge
    C. The most important drug
    D. The solid drug
28. You are giving a person tablets and capsules. You do all the following *except*
    A. identify the person
    B. provide for privacy
    C. let the person drink a small amount of water before taking a drug
    D. tell the person to hurry
29. Which statement about a sublingual drug is *true*?
    A. It is placed under the tongue.
    B. It is also called a buccal tablet.
    C. The person should drink water with it.
    D. It is placed between the upper molar and the cheek.

Fill in the Blanks
For questions 30-32 write out the meaning of each abbreviation.

30. GI _____

    _____

31. ISMP _____

    _____

32. PO _____

    _____

33. A syrup contains drugs dissolved in _____

    _____ .

34. Place a container cap _____ on a clean surface.

35. Buccal tablets are placed between the _____ and the molar teeth.

True/False
Circle T if the statement is true. Circle F if the statement is false.

36. T   F   When giving a crushed drug with food, the person must ingest all the food the drug is mixed with.

37. T   F   To divide a dose, you may break a tablet that is scored.

38. T   F   Lozenges are held in the mouth so they dissolve slowly.

39. T   F   Before giving a suspension, you shake the bottle.

40. T   F   Lozenges are commonly called "cough drops."

41. T   F   When giving drugs, you should use terms that the person can understand.

42. T   F   A medicine cup is accurate for doses larger than 1 teaspoon.

43. T   F   You are in a person's home. The person is to receive 2 teaspoons of a drug. You may use a kitchen spoon for measuring the drug.

44. T   F   When giving a drug using a syringe, you may use a parenteral syringe.

45. T   F   When giving a drug, you must follow the Six Rights of Drug Administration.

46. T   F   When giving a drug, you follow procedures to prevent infection.

47. T   F   Lozenges may be swallowed whole.

48. T   F   A person is to receive two liquid drugs. You may mix them together when you give them.

49. T   F   You are giving a capsule and cough syrup. You should give the cough syrup as the first drug.

50. T   F   You may return extra liquid that has been poured into a medicine cup back into the bottle.

51. T   F   You may mix a crushed tablet with food if directed by the nurse or MAR.

Labeling

52. You are to give ¼ oz of a drug. Mark with an "X" this amount on the medicine cup.

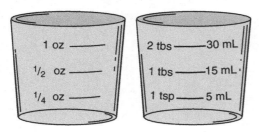

53. You are to give 15 mL of a drug. Mark with an "X" this amount on the medicine cup.

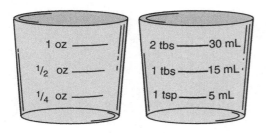

54. You are to give 1.5 mL of a drug. Mark with an "X" this amount on the medicine dropper.

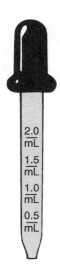

55. You are to give 2 mL of a drug. Mark with an "X" this amount on the oral syringe.

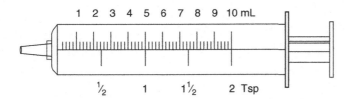

56. Label the parts of the oral syringe.

A _____

B _____

C _____

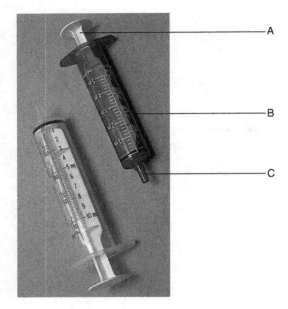

Independent Learning Activities

• Ask the instructor to show you the following drug forms used in your agency: capsules, tablets, lozenges, elixirs, emulsions, suspensions, and syrups.
• Look at souffle cups, medicine cups, medicine droppers, teaspoons, and oral syringes.
• Practice crushing a tablet.
• Practice taking a capsule apart.
• Role-play giving and documenting an oral drug in solid form.
• Role-play giving and documenting an oral drug in liquid form.
• Role-play giving and documenting a sublingual drug and a buccal drug.
• Role-play giving a capsule to a patient who is having difficulty swallowing.

11 Topical Drugs

Fill in the Blanks: Key Terms
Use these terms to complete questions 1–8.

Cream   Lotion   Powder   Topical medication
Debride   Ointment   Topical   Transdermal

1. A watery preparation containing suspended particles is _____.

2. A drug applied to the skin is a _____.

3. _____ means to remove.

4. A finely ground drug in a talc base is _____.

5. _____ means through the skin.

6. A semi-solid emulsion containing a drug is a _____
_____.

7. _____ refers to a surface of a part of the body.

8. A semi-solid preparation containing a drug in an oily base is an _____.

Circle the BEST Answer

9. You are applying a lotion. You should
   A. shake all lotions before the application
   B. rub the lotion onto the skin
   C. apply the lotion with an ungloved hand
   D. let the lotion touch your skin
10. When applying a topical drug, you do all the following *except*
    A. practice hand hygiene before and after the application
    B. wear gloves
    C. document before you apply the drug
    D. apply the dose form to clean, dry skin
11. To safely apply powder, you
    A. sprinkle a small amount of powder onto your hands or a cloth
    B. apply the powder in a thick layer
    C. let the powder fall on the floor
    D. shake powder onto the person
12. Before applying a topical drug, you should
    A. provide for privacy
    B. keep doors and window coverings open
    C. expose the person's body
    D. treat the person rudely

13. When applying nitroglycerin ointment, you do all the following *except*
    A. apply the drug to clean, dry skin that has little or no hair
    B. let the ointment touch your skin
    C. wear gloves
    D. remove the old application before applying a new one.
14. You are applying a transdermal patch. You
    A. cover the patch with a see through dressing
    B. remove the old transdermal patch before applying the new patch
    C. tell the person the drug is absorbed quickly
    D. apply a new transdermal patch before removing the old transdermal patch

Fill in the Blanks
For question 15 write out the meaning of the abbreviation.

15. TDD _____
_____

16. An _____ contains small droplets of water-in-oil or oil-in-water.

17. Drugs are applied topically to
    A. clean and _____ a wound
    B. hydrate (add water) the _____
    _____
    C. reduce _____
    _____
    D. relieve itching or a _____
    _____
    E. provide a protective _____ to the skin
    F. reduce thickening of the _____
    _____

True/False
Circle T if the statement is true. Circle F if the statement is false.

18. T   F   The absorption of a topical drug is affected by the amount of water in the tissues.

19. T   F   Wounds may be debrided with topical drugs.

20. T   F   Ointments are easily removed with water.

21. T   F   Standard Precautions are followed when you apply a lotion.

22. T   F   Before applying a topical drug, you clean and dry the skin.

23. T   F   A sterile tongue blade is used to remove a topical drug from a jar.

24. T   F   Before applying a topical drug to an older person, you ask the nurse what cleansing agent to use.

25. T   F   Before applying a topical drug, the nurse will tell you if isolation precautions are required.

26. T   F   Before applying a topical drug, the nurse will tell you if you need to cover the application.

27. T   F   You do not need to follow the Six Rights of Drug Administration when applying topical drugs.

28. T   F   When applying nitroglycerin ointment, the dosage applied must be accurate.

29. T   F   You may apply nitroglycerin ointment to irritated or open skin areas.

30. T   F   When applying nitroglycerin ointment, you rotate the application site.

31. T   F   When applying nitroglycerin ointment, you rub or massage the ointment into the skin.

32. T   F   Transdermal drug delivery system (TDD) provides continuous, gradual absorption of a drug through the skin and into the bloodstream.

33. T   F   When applying a topical drug, you observe for drainage or bleeding from wounds or body openings.

Independent Learning Activities

- Ask your instructor to show you creams, lotions, ointments, and powders used in your agency.
- Role-play applying creams, lotions, ointments, and powders.
- Role-play applying nitroglycerin ointment.
- Role-play applying a transdermal patch.

12 Eye, Ear, Nose, and Inhaled Drugs

Fill in the Blanks: Key Terms
Use these terms to complete questions 1–5.

Cerumen   Nasal   Ophthalmic
Instill   Ocular   Otic

1. Another term for nose is _____.

2. Two terms that pertain to the eye are _____ and _____.

3. _____ is another term for ear wax.

4. To enter drop by drop is to _____.

5. A term that pertains to the ear is _____.

Circle the BEST Answer

6. Ocular drugs are given in the
   A. nose
   B. mouth
   C. ear
   D. eye

7. When giving an eye or ear medication, you
   A. give an expired drug
   B. follow Standard Precautions
   C. let the dropper touch the eye or ear
   D. use the same bottle for different people

8. When giving an eye medication, you
   A. tilt the person's head forward
   B. remove eye secretions by cleaning from the outer to the inner aspect of the eye
   C. give eye drops at room temperature
   D. apply the drops or ointment to the cornea

9. The drug order has the abbreviation "OU." You should
   A. give the drug in the right eye
   B. give the drug in the left eye
   C. check with the nurse
   D. give the drug in both eyes

10. When applying eye drops, you do the following *except*
    A. give the eye drops in the dining room
    B. identify the person
    C. ask the person to look up toward the ceiling
    D. apply gentle pressure to the inner corner of the eyelid for 1 to 2 minutes

11. When giving ear drops, you
    A. give the drug order with the abbreviation AD
    B. insert cotton-tipped applicators into the ear
    C. remove cerumen you can see
    D. keep the ear drops refrigerated until needed

12. You are applying ear drops. You do the following *except*
    A. ask the person to remain in the side-lying position after receiving the ear drops for 5 to 10 minutes
    B. check with the nurse before inserting a cotton plug into the ear
    C. report and record redness, irritation, drainage
    D. ignore complaints of pain or discomfort

13. When giving an ear medication, you
    A. give the drug labeled *otic*
    B. document before giving the drug
    C. give a drug that is expired
    D. give the drug with visitors present

14. To apply ear drops to a person 3 years of age and older, you
    A. pull the ear upward and back
    B. pull the ear down and back
    C. pull the ear down and forward
    D. instill the drops without pulling the ear

15. When giving nasal medications, you
    A. explain that the medication may cause a burning or stinging feeling
    B. instill 2 drops of the drug
    C. hold the dropper about 1 inch above the nostril
    D. ask the person to blow his or her nose after receiving the medication

16. When using an MDI without a spacer, you do the following *except*
    A. shake the inhaler the number of times as directed by the nurse
    B. place the inhaler 1 to 2 inches in front of the person's mouth
    C. squeeze the dispensing valve and ask the person to inhale deeply and slowly for 3 to 5 seconds
    D. ask the person to hold his or her breath for about 30 seconds before exhaling slowly

Fill in the Blanks
For questions 17-18 write out the meaning of the abbreviations.

17. ISMP _____

_____

18. MDI _____

_____

True/False

Circle T if the statement is true. Circle F if the statement is false.

19. T   F   When giving eye medication, you apply the drug directly onto the eyeball.

20. T   F   After giving eye medication, you should use a tissue to blot medication that runs out of the eye.

21. T   F   You are giving an eye medication. It is labeled *ophthalmic*. You may give the drug.

22. T   F   You follow the Six Rights of Drug Administration when giving eye and ear drugs.

23. T   F   Cold eardrops can cause nausea, pain, and dizziness.

24. T   F   When giving nose drops, hold the dropper about ½ inch above the nostril.

25. T   F   Inhaled drugs have a rapid absorption rate and onset of action.

26. T   F   Before giving an MDI, you need to be sure your state and agency allows you to give the drug.

27. T   F   Before using an MDI, you should check the expiration date.

28   T   F   Manufacturer's instructions should be followed for meter-dosed inhalers.

Independent Learning Activities

• Role-play giving or applying eye drops, eye ointment, ear drops, nose drops, nasal spray, a meter-dosed inhaler without a spacer, and a meter-dosed inhaler with a spacer. Role-play documenting each of the drugs you give.

13 Vaginal and Rectal Drugs

Fill in the Blanks: Key Terms
Use these terms to complete questions 1–2.

Gynecologic   Suppository

1. A cone-shaped, solid drug that is inserted into a body opening and melts at body temperature is a

   _____.

2. A term that pertains to diseases of the female reproductive organs and breasts is _____.

Circle the BEST Answer

3. Vaginal drugs are
   A. given to treat gynecologic disorders
   B. smaller than rectal suppositories
   C. more square than rectal suppositories
   D. given to treat constipation and hemorrhoids

4. After receiving a vaginal drug, a woman should
   A. remain supine with her hips elevated for 5 to 10 minutes
   B. lie on her left side
   C. lie on her right side
   D. walk around as desired

5. Vaginal drugs are often given
   A. before the shower
   B. in the early afternoon
   C. at bedtime
   D. in the late afternoon

6. When giving a vaginal drug, you do the following *except*
   A. insert a suppository as far as possible into the vagina
   B. check the drug for an expiration date
   C. place the person in Fowler's position
   D. lubricate the applicator tip or suppository with water-soluble lubricant

7. Before giving a rectal drug, you
   A. place the person in the supine position
   B. ask the person to have a bowel movement
   C. ask the person to drink water
   D. place the person in the lithotomy position

8. When would you give a rectal drug?
   A. After recent prostate surgery
   B. After recent rectal surgery
   C. After a breast biopsy
   D. After recent rectal trauma

9. When giving a rectal suppository, you do the following *except*
   A. lubricate the suppository
   B. place the person in the Sims' position
   C. place the rounded tip of the suppository into the anus and rectum
   D. place the person in a prone position

10. A rectal drug is inserted
    A. about 1 inch into the rectum
    B. with an enema tube
    C. with an applicator
    D. about 2 inches into the rectum

True/False
Circle T if the statement is true. Circle F if the statement is false.

11. T   F   The site of action for a vaginal suppository is in the rectum.

12. T   F   Suppositories are stored in a cool place to prevent softening.

13. T   F   Some women prefer to self-administer vaginal drugs.

14. T   F   To give a vaginal drug, place the woman in a lithotomy position.

15. T   F   Rectal drugs are given if a person has diarrhea.

16. T   F   Vaginal suppositories are given at room temperature.

17. T   F   A woman should void before a vaginal suppository is given.

18. T   F   Gloves are worn when giving a rectal drug.

19. T   F   A rectal suppository may be inserted into feces.

20 T   F   A gloved index finger may be used to insert a vaginal suppository.

Independent Learning Activities
- Role-play giving a vaginal suppository on a mannequin.
- Role-play giving a vaginal cream with an applicator on a mannequin.
- Role-play giving a rectal suppository on a mannequin.

Drugs Affecting the Nervous System

Fill in the Blanks: Key Terms
Use these terms to complete questions 1–14.

Adrenergic fibers
Adrenergic blocking agent
Agonist
Anti-cholinergic agent
Barbiturate

Cholinergic fibers
Homeostasis
Hypnotic
Inhibitor
Insomnia

Neuron
Neurotransmitter
Sedative
Synapse

1. A chemical substance that transmits nerve impulses is _____.

2. A constant internal environment is _____.

3. A drug that inhibits adrenergic effects is an _____

   _____.

4. _____ are nerve endings that release acetylcholine (a neurotransmitter).

5. The _____ is the basic nerve cell of the nervous system.

6. A _____ is the junction between one neuron and the next.

7. A drug that produces sleep is a _____.

8. _____ are nerve endings that release the norepinephrine (a neurotransmitter).

9. An _____ is a drug that prevents or restricts a certain action.

10. A _____ is a drug that quiets the person; it gives a feeling of relaxation and rest.

11. A drug that acts on a certain type of cell to produce a predictable response is an _____.

12. A drug that depresses the central nervous system, respirations, blood pressure, and temperature is a

    _____.

13. _____ is a chronic condition in which the person cannot sleep or stay asleep all night.

14. A drug that blocks or inhibits cholinergic activity is an

    _____.

Circle the BEST Answer
15. The nervous system
    A. controls, directs, and coordinates body functions
    B. consists of the central nervous system
    C. controls laughter
    D. controls crying
16. Which is *not* a main part of the brain?
    A. cerebrum
    B. myelin sheath
    C. cerebellum
    D. brainstem

17. The cerebrum is
    A. the smallest part of the brain
    B. the center of thought and intelligence
    C. divided into three hemispheres
    D. controls dreams
18. What part of the brain regulates and coordinates body movements?
    A. cerebellum
    B. cerebrum
    C. brainstem
    D. myelin sheath
19. What part of the brainstem controls heart rate, breathing, blood vessel size, swallowing, coughing, and vomiting?
    A. midbrain
    B. pons
    C. medulla
    D. spinal cord
20. Which statement about the autonomic nervous system is *false*?
    A. It controls involuntary muscles.
    B. It controls heartbeat, blood pressure, intestinal contractions, and sweating.
    C. It is divided into the sympathetic nervous system and the parasympathetic nervous system.
    D. It controls voluntary muscles.
21. The autonomic nervous system has two major neurotransmitters. One is norepinephrine, and the other is
    A. neuron
    B. synapse
    C. cholinergic fibers
    D. acetylcholine
22. A person is scheduled to receive terbutaline (Brethine), an adrenergic drug. The person has tremors and orthostatic hypotension. You
    A. give the drug as ordered
    B. tell the nurse and record your findings
    C. skip the dose
    D. call the physician
23. Albuterol (Proventil) is used for asthma and emphysema because it is
    A. a sedative
    B. a bronchodilator
    C. an anti-convulsant
    D. a vasoconstrictor

24. Beta blocking agents are used to treat
    A. angina
    B. shock
    C. bronchitis
    D. emphysema
25. Before giving a beta blocker, you
    A. measure blood pressure, heart rate, and heart rhythm
    B. measure temperature
    C. measure radial pulse
    D. ask the person to rate his abdominal pain
26. Which drug is *not* a beta blocker?
    A. propranolol (Inderal)
    B. metaproterenol (Alupent)
    C. acebutolol (Sectral)
    D. metoprolol (Lopressor)
27. Cholinergic agents are used to diagnose and treat
    A. diabetes
    B. heart failure
    C. stroke
    D. myasthenia gravis
28. The generic name for Mytelase is
    A. urecholine
    B. ambenonium
    C. neostigmine
    D. mestinon
29. Before giving an anti-cholinergic agent, you
    A. measure blood pressure and heart rate
    B. measure temperature
    C. ask the person about eye pain
    D. measure radial pulse
30. Anti-cholinergic agents are used to treat all the following *except*
    A. gastro-intestinal disorders
    B. myasthenia gravis
    C. eye disorders
    D. Parkinson's disease
31. Which drug is *not* an anti-cholinergic agent?
    A. atropine (Atropine Sulfate)
    B. belladonna (Belladonna Tincture)
    C. bethanechol (Urecholine)
    D. propantheline (Pro-Banthine)
32. Sedative-hypnotics are used for all the following *except*
    A. to treat insomnia and improve sleep
    B. to decrease anxiety level
    C. to treat peptic ulcers
    D. to increase relaxation
33. A person is taking a sedative-hypnotic drug. You should
    A. record the person's intake and output
    B. observe the person's level of alertness and ability to perform motor functions
    C. monitor what the person eats
    D. check the person's blood glucose level
34. Barbiturate drugs can cause drowsiness, lethargy, headache, muscle or joint pain, and
    A. increased appetite
    B. increased temperature
    C. mental depression
    D. decreased blood sugar
35. When giving a barbiturate, you assist the nurse by doing the following *except*
    A. take an order to discontinue the drug
    B. measure pulse, respirations, and blood pressure
    C. observe the person's level of alertness
    D. ask the person about pain or discomfort
36. A person who is taking a barbiturate drug has problems with coordination. You
    A. discontinue the drug
    B. have the person walk alone
    C. assist the person with walking as needed
    D. tell the dietitian
37. A person complains of lethargy. You know this means the person
    A. has pain
    B. is anxious
    C. feels sleepy or drowsy
    D. is restless
38. A person taking butabarbital (Butisol) develops a rash. You
    A. give the next dose
    B. tell the nurse
    C. tell the person the rash is temporary
    D. call the doctor
39. Benzodiazepines can cause drowsiness, hangover, sedation, and
    A. excitement
    B. pain
    C. lethargy
    D. increased appetite
40. Why would a person receive flurazepam (Dalmane)?
    A. to decrease muscle pain
    B. to prevent convulsions
    C. to decrease anxiety
    D. to treat insomnia
41. Which statement about diphenhydramine (Benadryl) is *false*?
    A. It is available over the counter.
    B. It is avaliable as an inhaler.
    C. It can be used for insomnia for up to 1 year.
    D. The usual adult dose is 25-50 mg at bedtime.
42. Zaleplon (Sonata) should be taken
    A. before breakfast
    B. before lunch
    C. before dinner
    D. before going to bed
43. Which drug used for Parkinson's disease is *not* a dopamine agonist?
    A. amantadine hydrochloride (Symmetrel)
    B. bromocriptine mesylate (Parlodel)
    C. carbidopa, levodopa (Sinemet)
    D. entacapone (Comtan)
44. Before giving amantadine hydrochloride (Symmetrel) you should
    A. measure temperature
    B. measure blood pressure in the supine and standing position
    C. measure apical rate
    D. measure radial pulse

45. Bromocriptine mesylate (Parlodel) is used to
    A. relieve rigidity and tremor
    B. decrease temperature
    C. increase appetite
    D. decrease blood pressure
46. You are giving a person carbidopa, levodopa (Sinemet CR). The drug
    A. must be taken with juice
    B. must be swallowed whole
    C. may be crushed
    D. may be chewed
47. Carbidopa, levodopa (Parcopa) ODTs are
    A. given with water
    B. given with milk
    C. placed on the tongue with food
    D. given with juice
48. Pramipexole (Mirapex) is given
    A. with food or milk
    B. on an empty stomach
    C. only with juice
    D. before getting out of bed
49. When giving ropinirole (Requip), you assist the nurse with assessment by measuring vital signs and
    A. reporting hallucinations, nightmares, or anxiety
    B. performing ADLs for the person
    C. giving the drug on an empty stomach
    D. ignoring side effects from the drug
50. Which statement about COMT inhibitors is *false*?
    A. Entacapone (Comtan) and (Stalevo) are COMT inhibitors.
    B. COMT inhibitors allow less dopamine to reach the brain.
    C. Diarrhea may develop 1 to 2 weeks after therapy is started.
    D. The person may have brownish-orange urine.
51. An anti-cholinergic agent may be given to a person with Parkinson's disease. These drugs reduce
    A. drooling and tremors
    B. stiff and rigid muscles
    C. slow movements
    D. stooped posture
52. The classic sign of Alzheimer's disease (AD) is
    A. gradual loss of short-term memory
    B. problems with words or names
    C. confusion
    D. inability to walk without help
53. Which drug is *not* used to treat Alzheimer's disease?
    A. donepezil (Aricept)
    B. terbutaline (Brethine)
    C. memantine (Namenda)
    D. galantamine (Razadyne)
54. Donepezil (Aricept) is used to
    A. prevent social isolation
    B. improve cognitive skills
    C. prevent delusions
    D. assist the person with walking

55. Memantine (Namenda) is given to treat
    A. very mild AD
    B. mild AD
    C. moderate to severe AD
    D. very severe AD
56. When giving galantamine (Razadyne) you
    A. measure vital signs and weight
    B. measure intake
    C. measure output
    D. check blood glucose

Fill in the Blanks
Write out the meaning of each abbreviation.

57. AD _____
58. CNS _____
59. COMT _____
60. g _____
61. GI _____
62. IM _____
63. IV _____
64. mcg _____
65. mg _____
66. mL _____
67. MI _____
68. mmHg _____
69. ODT _____

Matching

Match the brand name of the adrenergic agent with its generic name.

70. _____ Proventil

71. _____ Alupent

72. _____ Neo-Synephrine

73. _____ Brethine

A. terbutaline
B. albuterol
C. phenylephrine
D. metaproterenol

Match the brand name of the beta-adrenergic agent with its generic name.

74. _____ Sectral

75. _____ Levatol

76. _____ Inderal

77. _____ Blocadren

A. timolol
B. propranolol
C. penbutolol
D. acebutolol

Match the brand name of the cholinergic agent with its generic name.

78. _____ Mytelase

79. _____ Urecholine

80. _____ Prostigmin

81. _____ Mestinon

A. neostigmine
B. pyridostigmine
C. ambenonium
D. bethanechol

Match the brand name of the anti-cholinergic agent with its generic name.

82. _____ Atropine sulfate

83. _____ Bentyl

84. _____ Robinul

85. _____ Pro-Banthine

A. propantheline
B. atropine
C. dicyclomine
D. glycopyrrolate

Match the brand name of the barbiturate agent with its generic name.

86. _____ Butisol

87. _____ Mebaral

88. _____ Nembutal

89. _____ Luminal

A. pentobarbital
B. phenobarbital
C. butabarbital
D. mephobarbital

Match the brand name of the benzodiazepine agent with its generic name.

90. _____ ProSom

91. _____ Dalmane

92. _____ Ativan

93. _____ Doral

94. _____ Restoril

95. _____ Halcion

A. triazolam
B. estazolam
C. temazepam
D. flurazepam
E. quazepam
F lorazepam

Match the brand name of the non-barbiturate, non-benzodiazepine agent with its generic name.

96. _____ Aquachloral

97. _____ Unisom

98. _____ Lunesta

99. _____ Ambien

A. zolpidem
B. chloral hydrate
C. doxylamine
D. eszopiclone

Match the brand name of the anti-cholinergic agent with its generic name.

100. _____ Cogentin

101. _____ Akineton

102 _____ Benadryl

103. _____ Banflex

A. benztropine mesylate
B. orphenadrine citrate
C. diphenhydramine hydrochloride
D. biperiden hydrochloride

True/False
Circle T if the statement is true. Circle F if the statement is false.

104. T   F   All nerve fibers have a protective covering called a myelin sheath.

105. T   F   Nerve fibers covered with a myelin sheath conduct impulses slower than those fibers without it.

106. T   F   The brain and spinal cord make up the central nervous system.

107. T   F   The cerebral cortex controls memory, speech, voluntary muscle movement, vision, hearing, and other activities.

108. T   F   The spinal cord contains pathways that conduct messages to and from the brain.

109. T   F   Cerebrospinal fluid protects the central nervous system.

110. T   F   The peripheral nervous system has cranial nerves and spinal nerves.

111. T   F   The autonomic nervous system controls the heartbeat and intestinal contractions.

112. T   F   When you are angry, scared, excited, or exercising, the parasympathetic nervous system is stimulated.

113. T   F   You may give a drug parenterally when asked by a nurse.

114. T   F   The autonomic nervous system maintains homeostasis.

115. T   F   Most organs have both adrenergic and cholinergic fibers.

116. T   F   Adrenergic agents stimulate the sympathetic nervous system.

117. T   F   Cholinergic agents stimulate the parasympathetic nervous system.

118. T   F   Before giving an adrenergic drug, the nurse may ask you to take the person's blood pressure and heart rate.

119. T   F   When a beta blocker is discontinued, the dose is reduced over 1 to 2 weeks.

120. T   F   Most body systems are affected by cholinergic fibers.

121. T   F   Adverse effects from cholinergic agents are not always seen.

122. T   F   Anti-cholinergic agents are also called cholinergic blocking agents.

123. T   F   An older person who takes a barbiturate may become restless or confused.

124. T   F   A person with "morning hangover" may have blurred vision or dizziness.

125. T   F   The habitual use of benzodiazepines may result in physical and psychological dependence.

126. T   F   Orthostatic hypotension is common with most drugs used to treat Parkinson's disease.

127. T   F   The classic sign of Alzheimer's disease is quick loss of long-term memory.

Independent Learning Activities
- Obtain index cards. On each card, write the name of a drug class, observations to make when giving drugs in this class, and what to report and record. Here is an example:
Drug Class: Adrenergic Agents
Observations:
Report and record:
- Make flash cards for each of the drugs in the following tables. Include the generic name of the drug, the brand name, dose, action, clinical use, and comments.
  - Adrenergic Agents—Table 14-1
  - Beta-Adrenergic Agents—Table 14-2

- Cholinergic Agents—Table 14-3
- Anti-Cholinergic Agents—Table 14-4
- Barbiturates Agents—Table 14-5
- Benzodiazepines Used for Sedation-Hypnosis—Table 14-6
- Non-Barbiturate, Non-Benzodiazepine Sedative-Hypnotic Agents—Table 14-7
- Anti-Cholinergic Agents Used to Treat Parkinson's Disease—Table 14-8
- Ask your instructor to tell you which of the drugs in Tables 14-1 through 14-8 are used in your agency. For each of these drugs, place a star on your drug card.

Drugs Used for Mental Health Disorders

Fill in the Blanks: Key Terms
Use these terms to complete questions 1–6.

Antagonist
Anti-anxiety drugs

Anti-depressants
Anxiety

Psychosis
Tranquilizers

1. A vague, uneasy feeling in response to stress is _____

    _____.

2. An _____ is a drug that exerts an opposite action to that of another; or it competes for the same receptor sites.

3. Anti-anxiety drugs are called _____.

4. Several classes of drugs used to treat mood disorders are _____.

5. _____ are drugs used to treat anxiety.

6. _____ is a state of severe mental impairment; the person does not view the real or unreal correctly.

Circle the BEST Answer

7. A person with a mental health disorder has problems coping or adjusting to
    A. diets
    B. stress
    C. abuse
    D. aging

8. Which mental health disorder is *not* an anxiety disorder?
    A. obsessive-compulsive disorder
    B. major depression
    C. phobias
    D. post-traumatic stress disorder

9. Signs and symptoms of anxiety may include all the following *except*
    A. slow pulse
    B. dry mouth
    C. poor attention span
    D. difficulty following directions

10. Post-traumatic stress disorder occurs
    A. before a harmful event
    B. after a harmful event
    C. only in adults
    D. only in children

11. A person is constantly washing his or her hands. This may indicate
    A. an obsessive-compulsive disorder
    B. a panic disorder
    C. a phobia
    D. a bipolar disorder

12. A person with a bipolar disorder
    A. has emotional lows and emotional highs
    B. is always depressed
    C. has intense fear
    D. is always manic

13. Schizophrenia is
    A. a chronic and disabling brain disorder
    B. an acute and disabling brain disorder
    C. an anxiety disorder
    D. a phobia

14. Which drug class is commonly used to treat anxiety disorders?
    A. benzodiazepines
    B. monoamine oxidase inhibitors
    C. anti-psychotic agents
    D. tri-cyclic anti-depressants

15. The most common side effects of benzodiazepines are
    A. anxiety and nervousness
    B. hypertension and increased pulse
    C. drowsiness and loss of coordination
    D. hunger and thirst

16. Which drug is *not* an anti-anxiety agent?
    A. buspirone (BuSpar)
    B. bupropion hydrochloride (Wellbutrin)
    C. fluvoxamine (Luvox)
    D. hydroxyzine (Vistaril)

17. A person is taking too much buspirone (BuSpar) if he or she has
    A. diarrhea
    B. constipation
    C. slurred speech and dizziness
    D. hypertension

18. Fluvoxamine (Luvox) is used to treat
    A. obsessive-compulsive disorder
    B. bipolar disorder
    C. major depression
    D. phobias

19. Hydroxyzine (Vistaril), (Atarax) are used for the following *except*
    A. to control itching from allergic reactions
    B. to prevent vomiting
    C. to decrease anxiety
    D. to decrease relaxation before surgery

20. Which drug class is *not* used for mood disorders?
    A. monoamine oxidase inhibitors
    B. tri-cyclic anti-depressants
    C. selective serotonin re-uptake inhibitors
    D. anti-psychotic agents

21. The most common side effect of monoamine oxidase inhibitors is
    A. depression
    B. phobia
    C. orthostatic hypotension
    D. increased thirst

22. Which drug is *not* an MAOI?
    A. phenelzine (Nardil)
    B. selegiline (Emsam)
    C. desipramine (Norpramin)
    D. tranylcypromine (Parnate)
23. A person taking isocarboxazid (Marplan) is allowed to have
    A. aged cheese
    B. salami, pepperoni, and sausage
    C. coffee
    D. red wine and beer
24. When giving MAOIs, you assist the nurse with assessment by doing all of the following *except*
    A. measure height and weight
    B. measure blood pressure in the supine and standing positions
    C. measure blood glucose
    D. ask about foods and fluids consumed during the past few days
25. The initial dose of phenelzine (Nardil) is
    A. 15 mg three times a day
    B. 30 mg twice a day
    C. 60 mg daily
    D. 6 mg four times a day
26. The last dose of an MAOI should be given
    A. before 1600
    B. before 1800
    C. before 2000
    D. before 2200
27. A person has been started on a selective serotonin re-uptake inhibitor (SSRI). You expect to see drug effects in
    A. 1 to 2 weeks
    B. 2 to 4 weeks
    C. 5 to 6 weeks
    D. 7 to 8 weeks
28. When giving SSRIs, you assist the nurse with assessment by doing the following *except*
    A. measure blood pressure in the supine and standing positions
    B. weigh the person monthly
    C. observe for insomnia, nervousness, and other CNS signs and symptoms
    D. ask the person about GI symptoms
29. You are giving a person an SSRI drug. To decrease GI effects, you give the drug
    A. before breakfast
    B. at bedtime
    C. between meals
    D. with food
30. Which statement about tri-cyclic anti-depressants is *false*?
    A. They produce anti-depressant and tranquilizing effects.
    B. After 2 to 4 weeks of therapy, they elevate mood and improve appetite.
    C. Some TCAs are also used to treat cancer pain and eating disorders.
    D. After 2 to 4 weeks of therapy, they decrease mood and appetite.

31. A person is taking a TCA. A common occurrence is
    A. constipation
    B. diarrhea
    C. urinary frequency
    D. bradycardia
32. Which statement about TCAs is *false*?
    A. Dose increases are usually started in the morning.
    B. The initial dose of amitriptyline is 25 mg three times daily.
    C. The maximum daily dose of Norpramin is 300 mg.
    D. The daily maintenance dose of Tofranil is 30 to 75 mg daily at bedtime.
33. Bupropion hydrochloride (Wellbutrin) is an
    A. anti-depressant
    B. anti-psychotic agent
    C. anti-anxiety agent
    D. anti-manic agent
34. A person is taking bupropion hydrochloride (Wellbutrin). You do all the following *except*
    A. give the drug between meals
    B. report and record restlessness, agitation, anxiety, and insomnia
    C. report and record seizures
    D. report and record suicidal actions
35. Which statement about maprotiline is *false*?
    A. Measure blood pressure in the supine, sitting, and standing positions.
    B. Weigh the person weekly.
    C. The usual maintenance dose is 150 mg daily.
    D. Dosage increases are usually made in the morning.
36. You are giving a person mirtazapine (Remeron). Which statement is *false*?
    A. It is a serotonin antagonist.
    B. You measure blood pressure in the supine, sitting, and standing positions.
    C. The nurse may ask you to weigh the person weekly.
    D. Dosage increases are usually made in the morning.
37. You are giving a person hefazodone. Which statement is *false*?
    A. It increases symptoms of depression.
    B. Observe for orthostatic hypotension.
    C. The normal dose range is 300 to 600 mg daily.
    D. Observe for CNS symptoms.
38. You are giving a person trazodone hydrochloride (Desyrel). Which statement is *false*?
    A. It reduces symptoms of depression.
    B. Dosage increases are usually made in the evening.
    C. Give the drug before a meal.
    D. Report tachycardia or an irregular pulse.
39. You are giving venlafaxine (Effexor). Which statement is *false*?
    A. It is used to treat depression and anxiety.
    B. You measure blood pressure and weight.
    C. You give it with food.
    D. You give it at bedtime.
40. Brand names for lithium are Eskalith and
    A. Prozac
    B. Luvox
    C. Lithane
    D. Zoloft

41. A person taking lithium must maintain a normal dietary intake of sodium and
    A. drink 10 to 12 glasses of water daily
    B. drink 2 to 4 glasses of water daily
    C. drink 5 to 6 glasses of water daily
    D. drink 6 to 8 glasses of water daily
42. When giving anti-psychotic drugs, you assist with the nursing process by doing the following *except*
    A. measure blood pressure in the supine, sitting, and standing positions
    B. measure weight and height
    C. measure blood glucose
    D. measure intake and output
43. Anti-psychotic drugs are given for
    A. phobias
    B. obsessive-compulsive disorder
    C. acute mania
    D. schizophrenia
44. Which drug is *not* a first generation anti-psychotic agent?
    A. chlorpromazine (Thorazine)
    B. prochlorperazine (Compazine)
    C. clozapine (Clozaril)
    D. fluphenazine (Prolixin)
45. Which statement about acamprosate (Campral) is *false*?
    A. It is used for chronic alcohol patients who want to maintain a sober state.
    B. The adult dose is two 333-mg tablets (666 mg) once a day.
    C. Diarrhea tends to resolve with continued therapy.
    D. Observe the person's level of alertness and orientation to person, time, and place.
46. A person is taking disulfiram (Antabuse). Which statement is *true*?
    A. The person may use sleep aids or cold products that contain alcohol.
    B. The person may use mouthwashes that contain alcohol.
    C. The person may eat sauces and other foods that contain alcohol.
    D. The drug is given after the person has not had alcohol for at least 12 hours.

Fill in the Blanks
Write out the meaning of each abbreviation.

47. CNS _____

48. GI _____

49. MAOI _____

50. mg _____

51. mL _____

52. OCD _____

53. PO _____

54. PTSD _____

55. SSRI _____

56. TCA _____

Matching
Match the brand name of the benzodiazepine drug with its generic name.

57. _____ Xanax
58. _____ Serax
59 _____ Valium
60. _____ Ativan
61. _____ Tranxene

A. oxazepam
B. alprazolam
C. clorazepate
D. diazepam
E. lorazepam

Match the brand name of the MAOI with its generic name.

62. _____ Nardil
63. _____ Parnate
64. _____ Marplan
65. _____ Emsam

A. selegiline
B. tranylcypromine
C. phenelzine
D. isocarboxazid

Match the brand name of the SSRI with its generic name.

66. _____ Celexa
67. _____ Cymbalta
68. _____ Lexapro
69. _____ Prozac
70. _____ Luvox
71. _____ Paxil
72. _____ Zoloft

A. sertraline
B. citalopram
C. paroxetine
D. duloxetine
E. fluvoxamine
F. escitalopram
G. fluoxetine

Match the brand name of the TCA with its generic name.

73. _____ Elavil
74. _____ Norpramin
75. _____ Sinequan
76. _____ Tofranil
77. _____ Aventyl, Pamelor
78. _____ Vivactil
79. _____ Surmontil

A. trimipramine
B. protriptyline
C. nortriptyline
D. imipramine
E. doxepin
F. desipramine
G. amitriptyline

Match the term with the appropriate example.

80. _____ Delusion
81. _____ Hallucination
82. _____ Paranoia
83. _____ Delusion of grandeur
84. _____ Delusion of persecution

A. A person believes others are cheating or plotting against him or her.
B. A person believes a radio station is broadcasting the person's thoughts.
C. A man believes he is Superman; a woman believes she is the Queen of England.
D. A person sees animals, insects, or people that are not real.
E. A person believes someone is "out to get" him or her.

True/False
Circle T if the statement is true. Circle F if the statement is false.

85. T F The person with a mental health disorder has problems adjusting to stress.
86. T F Panic is the lowest level of anxiety.
87. T F A person with aquaphobia fears being trapped in an enclosed space.
88. T F Bipolar disorder is also called manic-depressive illness.
89. T F Older persons do not become depressed.
90. T F Many of the drugs used to treat mental health disorders affect the CNS.
91. T F Anti-anxiety drugs are also known as tranquilizers.
92. T F Mood disorders involve feelings, emotions, and moods.
93. T F Mood disorders are also called affective disorders.
94. T F Older persons are often diagnosed as having dementia instead of depression.
95. T F Anti-depressants may decrease the risk of suicidal thinking and behavior.
96. T F MAOIs can cause serious hypertension if taken with foods or fluids that contain tyramine.
97. T F Constipation is a common side effect with TCA drugs.
98. T F Lithium is given with food or milk.
99. T F Schizophrenia is the most common psychotic disorder.

100. T   F   Typical anti-psychotic agents may also be called first-generation anti-psychotic agents.

101. T   F   Atypical anti-psychotic agents may also be called second-generation anti-psychotic agents.

102. T   F   Anti-psychotic drugs have few adverse effects.

Independent Learning Activities

- Obtain index cards. On each card, write the name of a drug class, observations to make when giving drugs in this class, and what to report and record. Here is an example:
  Drug Class: Benzodiazepines
  Observations:
  Report and record:
- Make flash cards for each of the drugs in the following tables. Include the generic name of the drug, the brand name, dose, action, clinical use, and comments.
  Benzodiazepines—Table 15-1
  Anti-Depressants—Table 15-2
  Anti-Psychotic Agents—Table 15-3
- Ask your instructor to tell you which of the drugs in Tables 15-1 through 15-3 are used in your agency. For each of these drugs, place a star on your drug card.

16 Drugs Used for Seizure Disorders

Fill in the Blanks: Key Terms
Use these terms to complete questions 1–3.

Anti-convulsants   Epilepsy   Seizure

1. A brain disorder in which clusters of nerve cells sometimes signal abnormally is _____.

2. _____ are drugs used to prevent or reduce seizures.

3. A convulsion may also be called a _____.

Circle the BEST Answer

4. All of the following may cause a seizure *except*
   A. diabetes
   B. high fever
   C. brain tumor
   D. drug overdose

5. Anti-convulsant therapy is the main treatment for
   A. hypertension
   B. urinary frequency
   C. seizures
   D. stroke

6. A person has a seizure that lasts a few seconds. There is loss of consciousness, twitching of the eyelids, and staring. This is a
   A. partial seizure
   B. generalized tonic-clonic seizure
   C. generalized absence seizure (petit mal)
   D. grand mal seizure

7. When giving benzodiazepines for anti-convulsant therapy, you observe the following *except*
   A. speech pattern
   B. degree of alertness
   C. orientation to person, time, and place
   D. food intake

8. The adult dosage range for clonazepam (Klonopin) is
   A. 300 mg/day
   B. up to 20 mg/day
   C. up to 90 mg/day
   D. 5 mg/day

9. A person who is taking a benzodiazepine must
   A. test his or her blood sugar daily
   B. monitor his or her blood pressure daily
   C. check his or her hearing yearly
   D. use caution around machines or when driving

10. When giving hydantoins, you assist the nurse by
   A. measuring blood glucose
   B. measuring blood pressure
   C. observing the person's urinary output
   D. measuring weight

11. The adult dosage range for phenytoin (Dilantin) is
   A. 2-3 g/day
   B. 300-600 mg/day
   C. 20 mg/day
   D. 90 mg/day

12. The generic name for Peganone is
   A. ethotoin
   B. clorazepate
   C. diazepam
   D. clonazepam

13. The generic name for Zarontin is
   A. methsuximide
   B. ethosuximide
   C. ethotoin
   D. diazepam

14. The adult dosage range for methsuximide (Celontin) is
   A. 900-1200 mg/day
   B. 1000-1250 mg/day
   C. 300-600 mg/day
   D. 200-300 mg/day

15. The generic name for Tegretol is
   A. carbamazepine
   B. valproic acid
   C. primidone
   D. gabapentin

16. A person is taking gabapentin (Neurontin) and an antacid. When will you give Neurontin?
   A. 1 hour before the antacid
   B. 2 hours before the antacid
   C. 2 hours after the antacid
   D. with the antacid

17. A person taking a sprinkled capsule should
   A. swallow the capsule whole
   B. place the capsule under his or her tongue
   C. chew the drug
   D. let the drug dissolve in his or her mouth

18. Which statement about zonisamide (Zonegran) is *false*?
   A. It is taken with or without food.
   B. It may be taken at bedtime.
   C. The person taking it should drink 6 to 8 glasses of water each day.
   D. It is used to treat grand mal seizures.

Fill in the Blanks
Write out the meaning of each abbreviation.

19. g _____

_____

20. kg _____

_____

21. mg _____

_____

22. mL _____

_____

Matching

Match the brand name of the drug with its generic name.

23. _____ Klonopin

24. _____ Tranxene

25. _____ Valium

    A. diazepam
    B. clonazepam
    C. clorazepate

Match the brand name of the drug with its generic name.

26. _____ Trileptal

27. _____ Luminal

28. _____ Mysoline

29. _____ Gabatril

30. _____ Topamax

31. _____ Depakene

32. _____ Zonegran

    A. tiagabine
    B. zonisamide
    C. oxcarbazepine
    D. phenobarbital
    E. valproic acid
    F. primidone
    G. topiramate

True/False

Circle T if the statement is true. Circle F if the statement is false.

33. T   F   You may give an anti-convulsant drug parenterally.

34. T   F   After long-term use, benzodiazepines are discontinued rapidly.

35. T   F   Hydantoins are given with food or milk.

36. T   F   Lamotrigine (Lamictal) is an antacid.

37. T   F   Levetiracetam (Keppra) is used in combination with other anti-convulsants to treat partial seizures.

38. T   F   Topiramate (Topamax) may be given to prevent migraine headaches.

39. T   F   Valproic acid (Depakene) is given with food or milk.

Independent Learning Activities

- Obtain index cards. On each card, write the name of a drug class, observations to make when giving drugs in this class, and what to report and record. Here is an example:
  Drug Class: Benzodiazepines
  Observations:
  Report and record:
- Make flash cards for each of the drugs in the following tables. Include the generic name of the drug, the brand name, dose, action, clinical use, and comments.
  Drugs Used for Anti-Convulsant Therapy—Table 16-1
- Ask your instructor to tell you which of the drugs in Table 16-1 are used in your agency. For each of these drugs, place a star on your drug card.

17 Drugs Used to Manage Pain

Fill in the Blanks: Key Terms
Use these terms to complete questions 1–7.

Analgesic   Opiate   Synthetic
Euphoria   Opium
Pain   Semi-synthetic

1. An _____ is a drug that contains opium, is derived from opium, or has opium-like activity.

2. A substance that is made, rather than naturally occurring, is _____.

3. A drug that relieves pain is an _____.

4. The milky substance from unripe poppy seed pods is
_____.

5. _____ is an exaggerated feeling or state of physical or mental well-being.

6. *Aches*, *hurts*, *discomfort*, and *sore* are all terms for
_____.

7. A natural substance that has been partially altered by chemicals is a _____.

Circle the BEST Answer
8. Which statement about pain is *false*?
   A. Pain is subjective.
   B. Pain is personal and differs for each person.
   C. Pain is a warning that there is tissue damage.
   D. Pain is objective.
9. Pain from a heart attack is often felt in the left chest, left jaw, left shoulder, and left arm. This is an example of
   A. acute pain
   B. radiating pain
   C. chronic pain
   D. phantom pain
10. Who decides if a person is having pain?
    A. the CNA
    B. the MA-C
    C. the nurse
    D. the person
11. A pain scale describes the
    A. location of the pain
    B. description of the pain
    C. intensity of the pain
    D. factors causing the pain
12. Who decides when to give a PRN pain drug?
    A. the physician
    B. the MA-C
    C. the nurse
    D. the person

13. A person taking an opiate agonist has constipation. You do the following *except*
    A. follow the care plan for fluid intake
    B. follow the care plan for the person's diet
    C. measure vital signs
    D. give stool softeners as ordered
14. The nurse tells you that a person has respiratory depression. This means the person has a respiratory rate of
    A. 12 per minute or less
    B. 14 per minute
    C. 16 per minute
    D. 18 per minute
15. A person taking an opiate-agonist is light-headed and dizzy. You provide for safety by putting the person in a
    A. prone position
    B. supine position
    C. Sims' position
    D. lateral position
16. You are going to give a person codeine (Codeine Sulfate) for pain. The order on the MAR is for 120 mg q4-6h. You
    A. give 120 mg
    B. ask the nurse about the dose
    C. give 60 mg
    D. call the physician
17. It is 12 noon. A person who received hydromorphone (Dilaudid) at 10 AM is asking for more pain medication. You
    A. give the drug early
    B. tell the person to wait until it is time
    C. ask the person if he or she is addicted to the drug
    D. tell the nurse
18. Salicylates have the following effects *except*
    A. analgesic effect
    B. anti-inflammatory effect
    C. mental sluggishness
    D. anti-pyretic effect
19. Which drug is *not* a salicylate?
    A. aspirin (Zorprin)
    B. hydromorphone (Dilaudid)
    C. diflunisal (Dolobid)
    D. choline salicylate (Arthropan)

20. Which statement about non-steroidal anti-inflammatory drugs is *false*?
    A. They are given to persons who are allergic to aspirin.
    B. They are known as "aspirin-like" drugs.
    C. They reduce fever.
    D. They relieve minor aches and pains from the common cold.
21. Non-steroidal anti-inflammatory drugs are given
    A. with food or milk
    B. before meals
    C. between meals
    D. at bedtime
22. The maximum daily dose for buprofen (Advil) is
    A. 300 mg
    B. 2400 mg
    C. 1000 mg
    D. 2000 mg
23. Acetaminophen (Tylenol) is used for all of the following *except*
    A. to relieve fever
    B. to relieve inflammation
    C. to relieve musculoskeletal pain
    D. to relieve headache
24. Which of the following is *not* a brand name of acetaminophen?
    A. Tylenol
    B. Datril
    C. Aleve
    D. Tempra
25. Propoxyphene (Darvon) is given
    A. before breakfast
    B. before lunch
    C. with food or milk
    D. at bedtime
26. Which statement about pentazocine (Talwin) is *false*?
    A. The adult oral dose is 200 to 300 mg every 3 to 4 hours.
    B. It is a controlled substance.
    C. Its generic name is pentazocine.
    D. Clamminess, dizziness, sedation, and nausea tend to occur with the first dose.

Fill in the Blanks
Write out the meaning of each abbreviation.

27. CNS _____

28. g _____

29. GI _____

30. h _____

31. MAR _____

32. mcg _____

33. mg _____

34. MI _____

35. mL _____

36. NSAID _____

37. PG _____

38. PO _____

39. PRN _____

40. STAT _____

41. q _____

Matching
Match the brand name of the opiate-agonist with its generic name.

42. _____ Codeine Sulfate

43. _____ Dilaudid

44. _____ Levo-Dromoran

45. _____ Roxanol

46. _____ Oxycontin

47. _____ Demerol

A. meperidine
B. codeine
C. oxycodone
D. hydromorphone
E. levorphanol
F. morphine

Match the brand name of the non-steroidal anti-inflammatory with its generic name.

48. _____ Motrin

49. _____ Indocin

50. _____ Orudis

51. _____ Naprosyn

52. _____ Celebrex

A. naproxen
B. celecoxib
C. indomethacin
D. ibuprofen
E. ketoprofen

True/False
Circle T if the statement is true. Circle F if the statement is false.

53. T F You should report complaints of pain to the nurse.

54. T F Reducing anxiety helps lessen pain.

55. T F Pain usually seems worse when the person is rested.

56. T F Pain often seems worse at night.

57. T F Adults must be alert to behaviors that signal a child's pain.

58. T F To some people, pain is considered a sign of weakness.

59. T F Pain is often ignored by some people.

60. T F Older persons may have increased pain sensations.

61. T F A person who normally moans and groans has become quiet and withdrawn. This person may have pain.

62. T F Vital signs may be normal with chronic pain.

63. T F Opiate receptors within the CNS control pain.

64. T F Morphine and heroin are opiates.

65. T F Most opiate agonists can produce addiction.

66. T F Opiate agonists are not considered controlled substances.

67. T F Opiate agonists may cause constipation and urinary retention.

68. T F Salicylates cause hallucinations, euphoria, or sedation.

69. T F Aspirin increases blood clotting.

70. T F Aspirin is given with food or milk or with large amounts of water.

71. T F Tinnitus and impaired hearing signal salicylate toxicity.

72. T F The usual adult oral dose for Tylenol is 325 to 650 mg every 4 to 6 hours.

Independent Learning Activities

- Determine whether your state and agency permit you to give controlled substances.
- Obtain index cards. On each card, write the name of a drug class, observations to make when giving drugs in this class, and what to report and record. Here is an example:

  Drug Class: Opiate Agents

  Observations:

  Report and record:
- Make flash cards for each of the drugs in the following tables. Include the generic name of the drug, the brand name, dose, action, clinical use, and comments.

  Opiate Agonists—Table 17-1

  Salicylates—Table 17-2

  Non-Steroidal Anti-Inflammatory Drugs—Table 17-3

  Selected Analgesic Combination Products—Table 17-4
- Ask your instructor to tell you which of the drugs in Tables 17-1 through 17-4 are used in your agency. For each of these drugs, place a star on your drug card.

18 Drugs Used to Lower Lipids

Fill in the Blanks: Key Terms

Use these terms to complete questions 1–5.

Cholesterol
Dyslipidemia
Hyperlipidemia
Lipids
Triglycerides

1. Another term for fats is _____.

2. An abnormality of one or more of the blood fats is
_____.

3. _____ are fatty compounds that come from animal and vegetable fats.

4. A waxy, fat-like substance found in all body cells is
_____.

5. Excess lipids in the blood is _____.

Circle the BEST Answer

6. LDL is called
   A. the "bad cholesterol"
   B. the "good cholesterol"
   C. a triglyceride
   D. a lipid

7. Dyslipidemia may be caused by all of the following *except*
   A. heredity
   B. a diet high in fat, cholesterol, carbohydrates, calories, and alcohol
   C. regular exercise
   D. age and gender

8. You are giving a bile acid–binding resin in a powdered form. What should you do?
   A. Give the drug before breakfast.
   B. Give the person dry powder to swallow.
   C. Mix the powder with 2 to 6 ounces of water, juice, or soup.
   D. Give the drug at bedtime.

9. A person is taking a bile acid–binding resin. He or she may
   A. crush or cut the tablet
   B. chew the tablet
   C. take the drug with meals
   D. limit water intake

10. When giving nicotinic acid (Niacin), you do the following *except*
    A. measure temperature
    B. ask the person about abdominal pain, nausea, and flatus
    C. give it with food
    D. report and record flushing, itching, rash, tingling, headache

11. Which are the strongest anti-lipemic drugs?
    A. Niacin
    B. Statins
    C. Fibric acids
    D. Bile acid–binding resins

12. Statins do all of the following *except*
    A. reduce LDL and lower total cholesterol levels
    B. reduce inflammation and blood clotting
    C. reduce risk factors for MI and stroke
    D. reduce HDL

13. The daily dose of atorvastatin (Lipitor) is
    A. 5 mg daily
    B. 10-40 mg daily
    C. 45-50 mg daily
    D. 50 mg daily

14. The maximum daily dose of fluvastatin (Lescol) is
    A. up to 20 mg at bedtime
    B. up to 40 mg at bedtime
    C. up to 60 mg at bedtime
    D. up to 80 mg at bedtime

15. Which drug is a fibric acid?
    A. lovastatin–niacin (Advicor)
    B. gemfibrozil (Lopid)
    C. rosuvastatin (Crestor)
    D. pravastatin (Pravachol)

16. The generic name for Tricor is
    A. gemfibrozil
    B. fenofibrate
    C. atorvastatin
    D. lovastatin

17. Gemfibrozil (Lopid) is given
    A. at bedtime
    B. 60 minutes after meals
    C. 30 minutes before the morning and evening meals
    D. 30 minutes before the morning meal

18. Fenofibrate (Tricor) is given
    A. at bedtime
    B. with meals
    C. 30 minutes before the morning and evening meals
    D. 30 minutes before the morning meal

19. The brand name for ezetimibe is
    A. Lasix
    B. Tylenol
    C. Zetia
    D. Omacor

20. A common side effect from anti-lipemic drugs is
    A. hypotension
    B. dizziness
    C. nausea and abdominal discomfort
    D. headache

Fill in the Blanks
Write out the meaning of each abbreviation.

21. CAD _____

_____

22. g _____

_____

23. HDL _____

_____

24. LDL _____

_____

25. mg _____

_____

26. MI _____

_____

27. TLC _____

_____

Matching
Match the brand name of the bile acid–binding resins with its generic name.

28. _____ Questran

29. _____ Colestid

30. _____ Welchol

A. colesevelam
B. colestipol
C. cholestyramine

Match the brand name of the statin with its generic name.

31. _____ Lipitor

32. _____ Lescol

33. _____ Mevacor

34. _____ Pravachol

35. _____ Crestor

36. _____ Zocor

37. _____ Caduet

38. _____ Advicor

39. _____ Pravigard

40. _____ Vytorin

A. fluvastatin
B. atorvastatin
C. simvastatin-ezetimibe
D. lovastatin
E. pravastatin-aspirin
F. simvastatin
G. pravastatin
H. rosuvastatin
I. atorvastatin-amlodipine
J. lovastatin-niacin

True/False
Circle T if the statement is true. Circle F if the statement is false.

41. T   F   Atherosclerosis occurs when fat builds up on the walls of arteries and arterioles.

42. T   F   Atherosclerosis is often called "hardening of the arteries."

43. T   F   CAD is a leading cause of death in the United States in men and women.

44. T   F   The higher the HDL level, the higher the risk of CAD.

45. T   F   Losing weight can lower LDL.

46. T   F   Anti-lipemic drugs are used to reduce fats in the blood.

47. T   F   When giving bile acid–binding resins, you assist the nurse by asking the person about abdominal pain, nausea, and flatus.

48. T   F   The maximum daily dose of cholestyramine (Questran) is 12 g.

49. T   F   Niacin is the generic name for nicotinic acid.

50. T   F   Statins should be given with grapefruit juice.

51. T   F   Fibric acids lower triglyceride and LDL levels.

52. T   F   Ezetimibe (Zetia) and Omacor are anti-lipemic drugs.

Independent Learning Activities

- Obtain index cards. On each card, write the name of a drug class, observations to make when giving drugs in this class, and what to report and record. Here is an example:

  Drug Class: Bile Acid–Binding Resins

  Observations:

  Report and record:
- Make flash cards for each of the drugs in the following table. Include the generic name of the drug, the brand name, dose, action, clinical use, and comments.

  Statins—Table 18-1
- Ask your instructor to tell you which of the drugs in Table 18-1 are used in your agency. For each drug, place a star on your drug card.

Fill in the Blanks: Key Terms

Use these terms to complete questions 1–9.

Aldosterone	Blood pressure	Hypertension
Angiotensin	Cardiac output	Pre-hypertension
Anti-hypertensive agents	Diuretic	Renin

1. Another term for high blood pressure is _____ _____.

2. A substance that causes vaso-constriction, increased blood pressure, and the release of aldosterone is _____.

3. The amount of blood pumped with each heartbeat is _____.

4. _____ occurs when the systolic pressure is between 120 and 139 mm Hg or the diastolic pressure is between 80 and 89 mm Hg.

5. A substance that causes the kidneys to retain sodium is _____.

6. A drug that promotes the formation and excretion of urine is a _____.

7. An enzyme that affects blood pressure is _____ _____.

8. Drugs that reduce blood pressure are _____.

9. _____ is the amount of force exerted against the walls of an artery by the blood.

Circle the BEST Answer

10. In which situation will the person's blood pressure be lowest?
    A. when responding to stress
    B. when exercising
    C. when lying down
    D. when standing

11. Which blood pressure is normal?
    A. 136/84
    B. 118/78
    C. 142/88
    D. 158/82

12. A person has a BP of 142/90. This is considered
    A. normal
    B. pre-hypertension
    C. hypertension
    D. hypotension

13. A person has a BP of 130/80. This is considered
    A. normal
    B. pre-hypertension
    C. hypertension
    D. hypotension

14. A person can change all of the following risk factors for hypertension *except*
    A. high-salt diet
    B. gender
    C. being overweight
    D. lack of exercise

15. When giving a beta blocker, you should
    A. take the apical pulse and BP
    B. take temperature and BP
    C. take the radial pulse and BP
    D. take respiratory rate and BP

16. A person on a beta blocker is having bradycardia and wheezing. You
    A. give the drug as ordered
    B. with-hold the next dose
    C. with-hold the next dose if the nurse tells you to
    D. ask the person if he needs the drug

17. ACE inhibitors
    A. increase BP
    B. increase muscle strength
    C. reduce BP
    D. decrease respirations

18. The initial dose of benazepril (Lotensin) is
    A. 20 mg once daily
    B. 10 mg once daily
    C. 25 mg once daily
    D. 4 mg once daily

19. Captopril (Capoten) is given
    A. 1 hour before meals
    B. 1 hour after meals
    C. at bedtime
    D. any time of the day

20. The maintenance dose of enalapril (Vasotec) is
    A. 4-8 mg daily
    B. 5-10 mg daily
    C. 10-40 mg daily
    D. 75-450 mg daily

21. A person on an angiotensin II receptor blocker (ARB) may develop hypotension. You do all of the following *except*
    A. check the person often until blood pressure is stable
    B. measure blood pressure in the supine and standing positions
    C. remind the person to rise quickly from a supine or sitting position
    D. have the person sit or lie down if symptoms develop

22. Which drug is *not* an angiotensin II receptor blocker (ARB)?
    A. candesartan (Atacand)
    B. eprosartan (Teveten)
    C. irbesartan (Avapro)
    D. benazepril (Lotensin)
23. Eplerenone (Inspra) is
    A. an angiotensin II receptor blocker
    B. an aldosterone receptor blocking agent
    C. a beta blocker
    D. a calcium ion antagonist
24. A person is taking a calcium ion antagonist. During the first week, he or she may have
    A. fatigue
    B. hypotension
    C. headache
    D. diarrhea
25. When giving alpha-2 agonists, you assist the nurse by doing all of the following *except*
    A. take respiratory rate
    B. take the blood pressure in the supine and standing positions
    C. observe for signs and symptoms of depression
    D. observe the person's sleep patterns
26. A person is on clonidine (Catapres-TTS). The transdermal patch is
    A. applied to a hairless area of intact skin
    B. changed every 14 days
    C. placed in the same site when changed
    D. applied to hairy area
27. A person is on guanadrel (Hylorel). Adverse effects include the following *except*
    A. orthostatic hypotension
    B. elevated temperature
    C. sedation and lethargy
    D. edema
28. The usual dosage range for guanethidine sulfate (Ismelin) is between
    A. 5 and 10 mg
    B. 15 and 20 mg
    C. 25 and 50 mg
    D. 55 and 60 mg

Fill in the Blanks

For questions 29-35 write out the meaning of each abbreviation.

29. ACE _____

_____

30. ARB _____

_____

31. g _____

_____

32. mg _____

_____

33. MI _____

_____

34. mmHg _____

_____

35. PO _____

_____

36. ACE inhibitors reduce blood pressure by affecting the _____ system.
37. Calcium ion antagonists also are called _____ _____ and _____.
38. A person was started on an alpha-1 blocker. Hypotension with _____, _____ _____, and _____ may occur within the 15 to 90 minutes after the first several doses.
39. The generic name of Apresoline is _____ _____.
40. The generic name of Loniten is _____ _____.

Matching

Match the brand name of the ACE inhibitor with its generic name.

41. _____ Lotensin
42. _____ Capoten
43. _____ Vasotec
44. _____ Monopril
45. _____ Prinivil
46. _____ Univasc
47. _____ Aceon
48. _____ Accupril
49. _____ Altace
50. _____ Mavik

A. ramipril
B. benazepril
C. trandolapril
D. captopril
E. quinapril
F. enalapril
G. moexipril
H. lisinopril
I. perindopril
J. fosinopril

Match the brand name of the calcium ion antagonist with its generic name.

51. _____ Norvasc

52. _____ Cardizem

53. _____ Plendil

54. _____ DynaCirc

55. _____ Cardene

56. _____ Procardia

57. _____ Sular

58. _____ Calan

A. nisoldipine
B. nicardipine
C. felodipine
D. diltiazem
E. amlodipine
F. isradipine
G. nifedipine
H. verapamil

Match the brand name of the alpha-1 adrenergic blocking agent with its generic name.

59. _____ Cardura

60. _____ Minipress

61. _____ Hytrin

A. prazosin
B. terazosin
C. doxazosin

Match the brand name of the central-acting alpha-2 agonist with its generic name.

62. _____ Catapres

63. _____ Wytensin

64. _____ Tenex

65. _____ Aldomet

A. guanabenz
B. methyldopa
C. clonidine
D. guanfacine

Match the brand name of the peripheral-acting adrenergic antagonist with its generic name.

66. _____ Hylorel

67. _____ Ismelin

68. _____ Serpasil

A. guanethidine sulfate
B. guanadrel
C. reserpine

True/False
Circle T if the statement is true. Circle F if the statement is false.

69. T F   Drug therapy is necessary if life-style changes control blood pressure.

70. T F   Once drug therapy is started, it may take months to control hypertension.

71. T F   Diuretics may be prescribed to treat hypertension.

72. T F   Beta-adrenergic blocking agents may also be called beta blockers.

73. T F   Angiotensin-converting enzyme inhibitors reduce blood pressure.

74. T F   Eplerenone (Inspra) is given with or without food.

75. T F   Calcium ion antagonists are used to treat hypertension, arrhythmias, and angina.

76. T F   Verapamil (Calan) is given with food.

77. T F   A person started on reserpine (Serpasil) may have nasal congestion.

78. T F   Hydralazine (Apresoline) and minoxidil (Loniten) are direct vaso-dilators.

Independent Learning Activities
- Obtain index cards. On each card, write the name of a drug class, observations to make when giving drugs in this class, and what to report and record. Here is an example:
  Drug Class: Diuretics
  Observations:
  Report and record:

- Make flash cards for each of the drugs in the following tables. Include the generic name of the drug, the brand name, dose, action, clinical use, and comments.

  Angiotensin-Converting Enzyme (ACE) Inhibitors—Table 19-1

  Angiotensin II Receptor Blockers (ARBs)—Table 19-2

  Calcium Ion Antagonists (Calcium Channel Blockers) Used to Treat Hypertension—Table 19-3

  Alpha-1 Adrenergic Blocking Agents—Table 19-4

  Central-Acting Alpha-2 Agonists—Table 19-5

- Ask your instructor to tell you which of the drugs in Tables 19-1 through 19-5 are used in your agency. For each drug, place a star on your drug card.

20 Drugs Used to Treat Dysrhythmias

Fill in the Blanks: Key Terms
Use these terms to complete questions 1–3.

Anti-dysrhythmic agents   Arrhythmia   Dysrhythmia

1. _____ means without a rhythm.

2. Drugs used to prevent or correct abnormal heart rhythms are _____.

3. An abnormal rhythm is called a _____.

Circle the BEST Answer

4. What structure sets the beat of the heart?
   A. atrio-ventricular node
   B. sino-atrial node
   C. Purkinje fibers
   D. bundle of His

5. The normal heart rate for an adult is between
   A. 50 and 70 beats per minute
   B. 80 and 120 beats per minute
   C. 60 and 100 beats per minute
   D. 100 and 110 beats per minute

6. Dysrhythmias that develop below the bundle of His are called
   A. heart blocks
   B. ventricular dysrhythmias
   C. supraventricular dysrhythmias
   D. premature atrial contraction

7. The nurse tells you the person has sinus tachycardia. This means
   A. the heart rate is slow
   B. the SA node sends out an impulse early
   C. the heart rate is rapid
   D. the conduction impulses start in the atria at a rapid rate

8. All of the following describe a block in the conduction system of the heart *except*
   A. first-degree heart block
   B. second-degree heart block
   C. third-degree heart block
   D. fourth-degree heart block

9. Asystole means
   A. the conduction impulse is created in the ventricles
   B. conduction impulses start from multiple sites in the ventricles
   C. some impulses from the SA node do not reach the ventricles
   D. no electrical activity occurs in the heart

10. Which drug does *not* prevent or correct abnormal heart rhythms?
    A. amiodarone hydrochloride (Cordarone)
    B. disopyramide (Norpace)
    C. prazosin (Minipress)
    D. procainamide hydrochloride (Procanbid)

11. Before giving an anti-dysrhythmic drug, you observe for the following *except*
    A. dyspnea and fatigue
    B. chest pain and edema
    C. hearing loss
    D. fainting and palpitations

12. When giving an anti-dysrhythmic drug, you do the following *except*
    A. measure blood pressure
    B. measure radial pulse for 1 minute
    C. measure apical pulse for 1 minute
    D. measure respirations

13. Which drug can affect urination?
    A. amiodarone hydrochloride (Cordarone)
    B. disopyramide (Norpace)
    C. flecainide acetate (Tambocor)
    D. mexiletine (Mexitil)

14. The usual dose for flecainide acetate (Tambocor) is
    A. 100 mg twice a day
    B. 150 mg twice a day
    C. 200 mg twice a day
    D. 250 mg twice a day

15. The usual dose for mexiletine (Mexitil) is
    A. 100 to 200 mg every 8 hours
    B. 200 to 400 mg every 8 hours
    C. 400 to 600 mg every 8 hours
    D. 600 to 800 mg every 8 hours

16. Which statement about moricizine (Ethmozine) is *false*?
    A. It is used to change ventricular dysrhythmias to normal sinus rhythm.
    B. The drug is given around the clock.
    C. The drug is given with food or milk.
    D. The usual adult dosage is between 100 and 200 mg daily.

Fill in the Blanks
For questions 17-29 write out the meaning of each abbreviation.

17. AV bundle _____

_____

18. AV node _____

_____

19. ECG _____

_____

20. g _____

_____

21. GI _____

     _____

22. mg _____

     _____

23. PAC _____

     _____

24. PAT _____

     _____

25. PVC _____

     _____

26. SA node _____

     _____

27. VF _____

     _____

28. V fib _____

     _____

29. VT _____

     _____

Fill in the Blanks

30. List the four structures in the heart wall that make up the conduction system.

    A. _____

    B. _____

    C. _____

    D. _____

31. If the normal electrical conduction system of the heart is disturbed, a person may have an abnormal

    A. _____

    B. _____

32. The SA and AV nodes depend on _____ ions for electrical conduction.

33. A person may describe palpitations as

    A. _____

    B. _____

Matching
Match the brand name of the drug with its generic name.

34. _____ Cordarone

35. _____ Norpace

36. _____ Tambocor

37. _____ Mexitil

38. _____ Ethmozine

39. _____ Procanbid

40. _____ Rythmol

A. amiodarone hydrochloride
B. propafenone
C. disopyramide
D. procainamide hydrochloride
E. flecainide acetate
F. moricizine
G. mexiletine

True/False
Circle T if the statement is true. Circle F if the statement is false.

41. T   F   The heart contracts during diastole.

42. T   F   The heart chambers fill with blood during systole.

43. T   F   Electrocardiograms record the electrical activity of the heart's conduction system.

44. T   F   Anti-dysrhythmic agents are used to prevent or correct abnormal heart rhythms.

45. T   F   Amiodarone hydrochloride (Cordarone) may cause existing dysrhythmias to worsen.

46. T   F   A person taking amiodarone hydrochloride (Cordarone) should use sunscreens and wear long-sleeved shirts.

47. T   F   Procainamide hydrochloride (Procanbid) is given in divided doses around the clock.

48. T   F   A person taking mexiletine (Mexitil) may have fine hand tremors.

49. T   F   Moricizine (Ethmozine) may cause euphoria in some people.

50. T   F   If a dose of propafenone (Rythmol) is missed, you should check with the doctor on what to do.

51. T   F   Diarrhea is common when a person is taking quinidine.

Independent Learning Activities

- Obtain index cards. On each card, write the name of a drug class, observations to make when giving drugs in this class, and what to report and record. Here is an example:

  Drug Class: Anti-dysrhythmic agents

  Observations:

  Report and record:

- Make flash cards for each of the following drugs. Include the generic name of the drug, the brand name, dose, action, clinical use, and comments.

  Cordarone

  Norpace

  Tambocor

  Mexitil

  Ethmozine

  Procanbid

  Rythmol

  Quinidine

- Ask your instructor to tell you which of the drugs listed above are used in your agency. For each drug, place a star on your drug card.

21 Drugs Used to Treat Angina, Peripheral Vascular Disease, and Heart Failure

Fill in the Blanks: Key Terms
Use these terms to complete questions 1–8.

Digitalization   Hemorrheologic agent   Intermittent claudication   Vaso-dilators
Fatty oxidase inhibitor   Inotropic agents   Platelet aggregation inhibitor   Vaso-spasm

1. A drug that reduces the oxygen needed by myocardial cells to cause muscle contractions is a _____ _____.

2. A sudden contraction of a blood vessel causing vaso-constriction is a _____.

3. _____ are drugs that stimulate the heart to increase the force of contractions.

4. A drug that prevents platelets from clumping together and causes vaso-dilation is a _____.

5. Giving a larger dose of digoxin for the first 24 hours and then giving the person a daily dose is called _____.

6. A pain pattern usually described as aching, cramping, tightness, or weakness in the calves that usually occurs during walking is called _____.

7. _____ are drugs that widen blood vessels to increase blood flow.

8. A drug that prevents the clumping of red blood cells and platelets is a _____.

Circle the BEST Answer

9. All of the following increase the heart's need for oxygen *except*
   A. exertion
   B. smoking
   C. rest
   D. a heavy meal

10. Nitrates relieve angina by
    A. constricting arteries and veins
    B. dilating coronary arteries
    C. increasing blood pressure
    D. decreasing blood pressure

11. The *most* common side effect of nitrates is
    A. hypotension
    B. headache
    C. nausea
    D. fainting

12. Isosorbide dinitrate (Isordil) tablets are given
    A. at bedtime
    B. with meals
    C. on an empty stomach
    D. after meals

13. A person has sublingual nitroglycerin tablets. The nurse should be told at once if the person does not obtain relief of chest pain within
    A. 5 minutes
    B. 10 minutes
    C. 25 minutes
    D. 15 minutes

14. Sustained-release nitroglycerin tablets are usually taken
    A. with breakfast
    B. before meals
    C. on an empty stomach every 8 to 12 hours
    D. at bedtime

15. A person has an order to be given the topical ointment form of nitroglycerin. You do the following *except*
    A. rotate application sites
    B. use a site that is irritated
    C. close the tube tightly
    D. store the tube in a cool place according to agency policy

16. To which site would you *not* apply a nitroglycerin transdermal disk?
    A. upper chest
    B. pelvis
    C. inner side of the upper arm
    D. scars, skin-folds, and wounds

17. A nitroglycerin transdermal disk has become partly dislodged. You
    A. tape the disk in place
    B. leave the disk as it is
    C. ask the nurse what to do
    D. tell the person to be careful

18. Before giving a beta blocker for angina, you measure the person's
    A. blood pressure in the supine and standing positions
    B. radial pulse
    C. apical pulse
    D. weight

19. ACE inhibitors are used to prevent
    A. congestive heart failure
    B. myocardial infarctions
    C. coronary artery disease
    D. peripheral vascular disease

20. Which statement about ranolazine (Ranexa) is *false*?
    A. It is a fatty oxidase enzyme inhibitor.
    B. Dizziness, headache, constipation, and nausea are side effects.
    C. It may be taken with or without meals.
    D. Tablets may be broken, crushed, or chewed.

21. Which statement about pentoxifylline (Trental) is *false*?
    A. It is a hemorrheologic agent.
    B. You should ask the person to rate his or her pain before giving the drug.
    C. The usual dose is 200 mg two times a day.
    D. It is used to treat intermittent claudication.
22. Which statement about cilostazol (Pletal) is *false*?
    A. It is a platelet aggregation inhibitor.
    B. It helps platelets clump together.
    C. It improves blood and oxygen supply to tissues.
    D. The dose is given 30 minutes before or 2 hours after breakfast and dinner.
23. A person is on digoxin (Lanoxin). You do all the following *except*
    A. measure the apical pulse for 1 minute before giving the drug
    B. give the drug after meals to reduce stomach irritation
    C. report and record signs and symptoms of digoxin toxicity
    D. measure the radial pulse for 30 seconds before giving the drug
24. Before giving digoxin (Lanoxin), you take the person's pulse. It is 58 beats per minute. You
    A. give the drug
    B. call the pharmacist
    C. hold the drug and follow agency policy
    D. hold the drug and tell the nurse at the end of the shift

Fill in the Blanks
For questions 25-35 write out the meaning of each abbreviation.

25. ACE _____

26. CAD _____

27. CHF _____

28. h _____

29. MAR _____

30. mg _____

31. MI _____

32. mL _____

33. PO _____

34. PVD _____

35. q _____

36. Another term for angina is _____.

37. The goals of nitrate therapy are to
    A. Relieve the _____ of angina during an attack
    B. Reduce the _____ and _____ of anginal attacks
    C. Increase _____ and _____ tolerance

38. Isosorbide mononitrate (Imdur) should not be _____ or _____.

39. Calcium ion antagonists are also called _____.

40. Peripheral vascular disease (PVD) involves the blood vessels in the _____ and _____.

Matching
Match the brand name of the nitrate with its generic name.

41. _____ Isordil

42. _____ Monoket

43. _____ Nitrostat

A. isosorbide mononitrate
B. nitroglycerin
C. isosorbide dinitrate

Match the brand name of the calcium ion antagonist with its generic name.

44. _____ Norvasc

45. _____ Cardizem

46. _____ Vascor

47. _____ Cardene

48. _____ Procardia

49. _____ Calan

A. nifedipine
B. amlodipine
C. bepridil
D. verapamil
E. nicardipine
F. diltiazem

Match the brand name of the vaso-dilator with its generic name.

50. _____ Vasodilan

51. _____ Pavagen TD

52. _____ Dibenzyline

A. isoxsuprine hydrochloride
B. papaverine hydrochloride
C. phenoxybenzamine hydrochloride

True/False

Circle T if the statement is true. Circle F if the statement is false.

53. T   F   Angina occurs when the heart needs more oxygen.

54. T   F   Sublingual nitroglycerin tablets should produce a slight stinging or burning sensation when taken.

55. T   F   Sublingual nitroglycerin tablets are stored in a clear plastic container.

56. T   F   A person who takes transmucosal nitroglycerin tablets may eat while the tablet is in place.

57. T   F   Before giving a beta blocker for angina to a person who has diabetes, the nurse may ask you to measure the person's blood glucose.

58. T   F   Verapamil (Calan) is given with food.

59. T   F   Before giving a vaso-dilator, you ask the person to rate his or her pain.

60. T   F   Congestive heart failure occurs when the heart is weakened and cannot pump normally.

61. T   F   Angiotensin-converting enzyme (ACE) inhibitors may be used for the treatment of CHF.

Independent Learning Activities

- Obtain index cards. On each card, write the name of a drug class, observations to make when giving drugs in this class, and what to report and record. Here is an example:
  Drug Class: Nitrates
  Observations:
  Report and record:
- Make flash cards for each of the drugs in the following tables. Include the generic name of the drug, the brand name, dose, action, clinical use, and comments.
  Nitrates—Table 21-1
  Calcium Ion Antagonists Used to Treat Angina Pectoris—Table 21-2
- Ask your instructor to tell you which of the drugs in Tables 21-1 and 21-2 are used in your agency. For each drug, place a star on your drug card.

22 Drugs Used for Diuresis

Fill in the Blanks: Key Terms
Use these terms to complete questions 1–3.

Ascites   Diuresis   Diuretic

1. The increased formation and excretion of urine is
   _____.

2. The abnormal accumulation of fluid in the peritoneal cavity is _____.

3. A _____ is a drug that promotes the formation and excretion of urine.

Circle the BEST Answer
4. The purpose of a diuretic is to
   A. increase the loss of water from the body
   B. decrease the excretion of sodium from the body
   C. decrease the loss of water from the body
   D. increase the excretion of calcium from the body

5. The goals of therapy for loop diuretics are the following *except*
   A. promote diuresis
   B. reduce edema
   C. improve symptoms related to excess fluid in tissues
   D. decrease diuresis

6. A person is taking bumetanide (Bumex). You would expect diuretic activity to begin
   A. 10 to 15 minutes after administration
   B. 30 to 60 minutes after administration
   C. 2 hours after administration
   D. 3 hours after administration

7. The diuretic activity for ethacrynic acid (Edecrin) lasts
   A. 1 to 3 hours
   B. 4 to 5 hours
   C. 6 to 8 hours
   D. 9 to 10 hours

8. A person taking a thiazide diuretic develops hives, rash, and itching. You
   A. give the next dose
   B. report the symptoms to the nurse
   C. call the doctor
   D. call the pharmacist

9. A person allergic to sulfonamides may also be allergic to
   A. ethacrynic acid (Edecrin)
   B. digoxin (Lanoxin)
   C. furosemide (Lasix)
   D. bumetanide (Bumex)

Fill in the Blanks
For questions 10–11 write out the meaning of each abbreviation.

10. mg _____
    _____

11. mL _____
    _____

12. Loop diuretics inhibit the re-absorption of _____
    and _____.

13. Bumetanide (Bumex) is given with _____
    or _____ to reduce stomach irritation.

14. Bumetanide (Bumex) is given before _____
    to prevent nocturia.

15. Potassium-sparing diuretics excrete _____
    but retain _____.

16. List symptoms a person who is dehydrated or has electrolyte imbalance might have.
    A. _____
    B. _____
    C. _____
    D. _____

Matching
Match the brand name of the loop diuretic with its generic name.

17. _____ Bumex

18. _____ Edecrin

19. _____ Lasix

20. _____ Demadex

A. torsemide
B. ethacrynic acid
C. bumetanide
D. furosemide

Match the brand name of the thiazide diuretic with its generic name.

21. _____ Naturetin

22. _____ Diuril

23. _____ Esidrix

24. _____ Enduron

A. methyclothiazide
B. chlorothiazide
C. bendroflumethiazide
D. hydrochlorothiazide

Match the brand name of the thiazide-related diuretic with its generic name.

25. _____ Hygroton

26. _____ Lozol

27. _____ Zaroxolyn

A. indapamide
B. metolazone
C. chlorthalidone

Match the brand name of the potassium-sparing diuretic with its generic name.

28. _____ Midamor

29. _____ Aldactone

30. _____ Dyrenium

A. triamterene
B. spironolactone
C. amiloride

True/False
Circle T if the statement is true. Circle F if the statement is false.

31. T   F   A person is on furosemide (Lasix). You should measure his or her blood pressure daily in the supine and standing positions.

32. T   F   A person is on torsemide (Demadex). You should report and record changes in alertness and orientation to person, time, and place.

33. T   F   Thiazide diuretics reduce blood pressure.

34. T   F   Amiloride (Midamor) is given at bedtime.

35. T   F   Spironolactone (Aldactone) may cause breast tenderness and menstrual irregularities in women.

Independent Learning Activities
- Obtain index cards. On each card, write the name of a drug class, observations to make when giving drugs in this class, and what to report and record. Here is an example:
  Drug Class: Loop Diuretics
  Observations:
  Report and record:
- Make flash cards for each of the drugs in the following tables. Include the generic name of the drug, the brand name, dose, action, clinical use, and comments.
  Thiazide Diuretic Products—Table 22-1
  Thiazide-Related Diuretics—Table 22-2
  Combination Diuretics—Table 22-3
- Ask your instructor to tell you which of the drugs in Tables 22-1 through 22-3 are used in your agency. For each drug, place a star on your drug card.

Drugs Used to Treat Thrombo-Embolic Diseases

Fill in the Blanks: Key Terms

Use these terms to complete questions 1–9.

Anti-coagulants
Anti-platelet agents
Embolus

Infarction
Ischemia
Platelet inhibitors

Thrombosis
Thrombo-embolic diseases
Thrombus

1. A decreased supply of oxygenated blood to a body part is _____.

2. An _____ is a small part of a thrombus that breaks off and travels through the vascular system until it lodges in a blood vessel.

3. Drugs that prevent arterial and venous thrombi are

   _____.

4. Another term for a blood clot is _____.

5. Drugs that prevent platelet aggregation (clumping) are _____.

6. A local area of tissue death is an _____.

7. The process of clot formation is _____.

8. Another term for platelet inhibitors is _____

   _____.

9. Disease associated with abnormal clotting within blood vessels is _____.

Circle the BEST Answer

10. To prevent thrombo-embolic diseases, a person should do the following *except*
    A. do leg exercises
    B. begin ambulation early after surgery
    C. stand or sit for prolonged periods
    D. wear thrombo-embolic (TED) hose

11. Aspirin is used to reduce the frequency of the following *except*
    A. arrhythmias
    B. TIA
    C. stroke
    D. MI

12. Ticlopidine (Ticlid) is given
    A. before meals
    B. with meals
    C. after meals
    D. at bedtime

13. A nurse asks you to give heparin. You
    A. give the dose
    B. refuse to give the dose
    C. ignore the request
    D. refuse to give the dose and tell the nurse why

14. Warfarin (Coumadin) inhibits the activity of
    A. vitamin B
    B. vitamin C
    C. vitamin D
    D. vitamin K

15. A person is on warfarin (Coumadin). You do the following *except*
    A. check for bleeding
    B. ask about GI symptoms
    C. give the dose only if the nurse instructs you to give it
    D. give the dose the person tells you to give

Fill in the Blanks

For questions 16-21 write out the meaning of each abbreviation.

16. GI _____

    _____

17. IV _____

    _____

18. mg _____

    _____

19. MI _____

    _____

20. TED hose _____

    _____

21. TIA _____

    _____

22. A person taking clopidogrel (Plavix) may have bleeding. You would report and record

    A. _____

    B. _____

    C. _____

    D. _____

    E. _____

23. Anti-coagulants are often called _____.

24. The generic name for Coumadin is _____

    _____.

Matching
Match the brand name of the platelet inhibitor with its generic name.

25. _____ Persantine

26. _____ Plavix

27. _____ Ticlid

A. clopidogrel
B. ticlopidine
C. dipyridamole

True/False
Circle T if the statement is true. Circle F if the statement is false.

28. T F   Platelet inhibitors are used to reduce venous clot formation.

29. T F   Aspirin inhibits platelet clumping and prolongs bleeding time.

30. T F   Aspirin is given with meals to prevent stomach irritation.

31. T F   When giving dipyridamole (Persantine), you measure blood pressure in the supine and standing positions.

32. T F   Anti-coagulants can dissolve an existing clot.

33. T F   Before warfarin (Coumadin) is given, the nurse checks laboratory prothrombin times.

Independent Learning Activities
- Obtain index cards. On each card, write the name of a drug class, observations to make when giving drugs in this class, and what to report and record. Here is an example:
Drug Class: Platelet Inhibitors
Observations:
Report and record:
- Make flash cards for each of the following drugs. Include the generic name of the drug, the brand name, dose, action, clinical use, and comments.
Aspirin
Persantine
Plavix
Ticlid
Coumadin
- Ask your instructor to tell you which of the drugs listed above are used in your agency. For each drug, place a star on your drug card.

Drugs Used to Treat Respiratory Diseases

Fill in the Blanks: Key Terms
Use these terms to complete questions 1–13.

Antihistamines
Antitussives
Broncho-dilators
Cilia
Cough suppressants

Decongestants
Expectorants
Histamine
Intra-nasal
Mucolytic agents

Rhinitis medicamentosa
Rhinorrhea
Tracheo-bronchial tree

1. _____ means within the nose.

2. Drugs that cause vaso-constriction of the nasal mucosa are _____.

3. Drugs that suppress the cough center in the brain are _____.

4. _____ are small hair-like structures that project outward from the surfaces of some cells.

5. Drugs that reduce the stickiness and thickness of pulmonary secretions are _____.

6. Another term for nasal discharge is _____.

7. A substance released in response to allergic reactions and tissue damage from trauma or infection is a _____.

8. Another term for antitussives is _____.

9. The _____ includes the trachea, bronchi, and bronchioles.

10. Drug-induced congestion is _____.

11. Drugs that liquify mucus to promote the ejection of mucus from the lungs and tracheo-bronchial tree are _____.

12. _____ are drugs that relax the smooth muscles of the tracheo-bronchial tree.

13. _____ are drugs that compete with released histamine for receptors sites in the arterioles, capillaries, and glands in mucous membranes.

Circle the BEST Answer
14. The drugs of choice for allergic rhinitis are
    A. antihistamines
    B. anti-inflammatory agents
    C. expectorants
    D. decongestants
15. Which statement about sympathomimetic nasal decongestants is *false*?
    A. They reduce nasal congestion.
    B. They ease breathing.
    C. Rhinitis medicamentosa is a risk from mis-use.
    D. They provide permanent symptom relief.

16. Antihistamines are more effective if taken
    A. before symptoms first appear
    B. when symptoms first appear
    C. after symptoms appear
    D. at any time
17. During the pollen season a person with an allergy takes an antihistamine. The drug will be more effective if taken
    A. 10 to 15 minutes before going outside
    B. 20 to 30 minutes before going outside
    C. 45 to 60 minutes before going outside
    D. 70 to 90 minutes before going outside
18. The *most* common side effect from antihistamines is
    A. sedation
    B. dry mouth
    C. blurred vision
    D urinary retention
19. The adult dosage range for diphenhydramine hydrochloride (Benadryl) is
    A. 5-10 mg daily
    B. 15-20 mg daily
    C. 25-50 mg twice daily
    D. 25-50 mg three or four times daily
20. The generic name for Nasalcrom is
    A. budesonide
    B. cromolyn sodium
    C. flunisolide
    D. mometasone
21. Before taking an intra-nasal cortico-steroid, the person should
    A. drink a glass of water
    B. clear his or her nasal passages of secretions
    C. dry his or her eyes
    D. chew gum
22. Which statement about potassium iodide (SSKI) is *false*?
    A. It reduces the thickness of mucus.
    B. It should be given with food or milk.
    C. It is used in the treatment of COPD.
    D. It is an antitussive agent.
23. Robitussin (guaifenesin) is
    A. an antitussive agent
    B. a broncho-dilator
    C. an expectorant
    D. a mucolytic agent

24. Robitussin CoughGels (a brand of dextromethorphan) are an
    A. antitussive agent
    B. broncho-dilator
    C. expectorant
    D. mucolytic agent
25. The generic name for Spiriva is
    A. atrovent
    B. antrovent HFA
    C. ipratropium bromide
    D. tiotropium bromide
26. A person is taking ipratropium bromide (Atrovent). With usual dosages broncho-dilation lasts for
    A. 2 to 3 hours
    B. 4 to 6 hours
    C. 7 to 8 hours
    D. 9 to 10 hours
27. The usual dose for tiotropium bromide (Spiriva) is
    A. 1 capsule daily
    B. 2 capsules daily
    C. 1 capsule twice a day
    D. 2 capsules twice a day
28. The generic name for Dilor is
    A. aminophylline
    B. dyphylline
    C. oxtriphylline
    D. theophylline
29. The generic name for Bronkodyl is
    A. aminophylline
    B. dyphylline
    C. oxtriphylline
    D. theophylline
30. A person uses an inhalant cortico-steroid. You observe for
    A. mouth infections
    B. tachycardia
    C. urinary retention
    D. tremors
31. Montelukast (Singulair) and zafirlukast (Accolate) are
    A. antihistamines
    B. anti-inflammatory agents
    C. anti-cholinergic agents
    D. anti-leukotriene agents
32. Xanthine-derivative broncho-dilating agents
    A. constrict the bronchi
    B. are also called xanthine-derivatives
    C. increase breathing effort
    D. are given on an empty stomach
33. Montelukast (Singulair) has been shown to reduce the following *except*
    A. broncho-constriction
    B. daytime asthma symptoms
    C. night-time awakening
    D. hypotension

Fill in the Blanks
For questions 34-44 write out the meaning of each abbreviation.

34. CO_2 _____

35. COPD _____
    _____
36. g _____
    _____
37. GI _____
    _____
38. h _____
    _____
39. kg _____
    _____
40. mcg _____
    _____
41. mg _____
    _____
42. mL _____
    _____
43. O_2 _____
    _____
44. PO _____
    _____
45. The respiratory system brings _____ into the lungs and removes _____ from it.
46. The nose warms, _____, and _____ _____ inhaled air.
47. The medical term for throat is _____
    _____.
48. The medical term for voicebox is _____
    _____.
49. The medical term for windpipe is _____
    _____.
50. Matter coughed up from the lungs is called _____
    or _____.
51. A person is taking a nasal decongestant. You would report and record
    A. _____
    B. _____
52. The _____ is the mucous membrane lining the inner surfaces of the eyelids and outer part of the sclera.
53. Intra-nasal cortico-steroids reduce rhinorrhea, rhinitis, _____, and _____.

54. Lower respiratory diseases are treated with _____ _____, _____, _____ ___, _____, and _____ _____.

55. Beta-adrenergic broncho-dilating agents are given to ease _____ and _____ wheezing.

Matching
Match the brand name of the nasal decongestant with its generic name.

56. _____ Pretz-D
57. _____ Adrenalin
58. _____ Privine
59. _____ Afrin
60. _____ Neo-Synephrine
61. _____ Sudafed
62. _____ Tyzine
63. _____ Otrivin

A. tetrahydrozoline
B. ephedrine
C. xylometazoline
D. epinephrine
E. pseudoephedrine
F. naphazoline
G. oxymetazoline
H. phenylephrine

Match the brand name of the antihistamine with its generic name.

64. _____ Astelin
65. _____ Zyrtec
66. _____ Chlor-Trimeton
67. _____ Tavist
68. _____ Clarinex
69. _____ Benadryl
70. _____ Allegra
71. _____ Atrovent
72. _____ Claritin
73. _____ Phenergan

A. cetirizine
B. clemastine fumarate
C. desloratidine
D. fexofenadine
E. loratadine
F. promethazine hydrochloride
G. ipratropium
H. diphenhydramine hydrochloride
I. chlorpheniramine maleate
J. azelastine

Match the drug type with what it does.

74. _____ Expectorant
75. _____ Antitussive agent
76. _____ Broncho-dilator
77. _____ Anti-inflammatory agent
78. _____ Mucolytic agent

A. Reduces inflammation
B. Liquifies mucus
C. Reduces the stickiness and thickness of pulmonary secretions
D. Suppresses the cough center in the brain
E. Relaxes the smooth muscles of the tracheo-bronchial tree

Match the brand name of the beta-adrenergic agonist with its generic name.

79. _____ Proventil
80. _____ Tornalate
81. _____ Primatene Mist
82. _____ Foradil
83. _____ Xopenex
84. _____ Alupent
85. _____ Maxair
86. _____ Serevent Diskus
87. _____ Brethine

A. formoterol
B. albuterol
C. terbutaline
D. bitolterol
E. salmeterol
F. epinephrine
G. levalbuterol
H. pirbuterol
I. metaproterenol

Match the brand name of the inhalant cortico-steroid with its generic name.

88. _____ QVAR

89. _____ Pulmicort

90. _____ AeroBid

91. _____ Flovent HFA

92. _____ Azmacort

A. flunisolide
B. beclomethasone dipropionate
C. triamcinolone acetonide
D. budesonide phosphate
E. fluticasone

True/False
Circle T if the statement is true. Circle F if the statement is false.

93. T F   Sinuses are hollow air-filled cavities that drain into the nasal cavity.

94. T F   Alveoli are tiny one-celled air sacs at the end of the bronchioles.

95. T F   Respiratory tract fluids come from glands that line the respiratory tract.

96. T F   Antihistamines reduce nasal congestion.

97. T F   Decongestants reduce nasal congestion.

98. T F   Anti-inflammatory agents are used to treat cold symptoms.

99. T F   Antihistamines are the drugs of choice for the treatment of allergic rhinitis and conjunctivitis.

100. T F   Antihistamines reduce rhinorrhea, tearing, eye itching, and sneezing.

101. T F   A side effect of codeine is constipation.

102. T F   Xanthine-derivatives constrict the bronchi.

103. T F   A person is taking a broncho-dilator by inhalation and a cortico-steroid inhalant. The broncho-dilator should be taken first.

Independent Learning Activities
- Review your state regulations and your job description to see if you are permitted to give drugs by nebulizer.
- Obtain index cards. On each card, write the name of a drug class, observations to make when giving drugs in this class, and what to report and record. Here is an example:
  Drug Class: Sympathomimetic Decongestants
  Observations:
  Report and record:
- Make flash cards for each of the drugs in the following tables. Include the generic name of the drug, the brand name, dose, action, clinical use, and comments.
  Nasal Decongestants—Table 24-1
  Antihistamines—Table 24-2
  Intra-Nasal Cortico-Steroids—Table 24-3
  Antitussive Agents—Table 24-4
  Broncho-Dilators—Table 24-5
  Inhalant Cortico-Steroids—Table 24-6
- Ask your instructor to tell you which of the drugs in Tables 24-1 through 24-6 are used in your agency. For each drug, place a star on your drug card.

25 Drugs Used to Treat Gastro-Esophageal Reflux and Peptic Ulcer Diseases

Fill in the Blanks: Key Terms

Use these terms to complete questions 1–12.

Antacids
Antagonist
Anti-spasmodic agents
Coating agents

Gastro-intestinal prostaglandins
Histamine
Histamine (H₂)-receptor antagonists
Peptic

Peptic ulcer
Prokinetic agents
Proton pump inhibitors
Ulcer

1. Drugs that block the action of histamine are

_____ .

2. A shallow or deep crater-like sore of a mucous membrane is an _____ .

3. Drugs that form a substance that adheres to the crater of an ulcer are _____ .

4. Drugs that buffer, neutralize, or absorb hydrochloric acid in the stomach are _____ .

5. _____ are drugs that inhibit the gastric acid pump of the parietal cells.

6. _____ pertains to the digestion or the enzymes and secretions needed for digestion.

7. Drugs that inhibit gastric acid secretion are

_____ .

8. _____ are drugs that have anti-cholinergic action and prevent acetylcholine from attaching to cholinergic receptors in the GI tract.

9. A substance released in response to allergic reactions and tissue damage from trauma or infection is a

_____ .

10. _____ are drugs that stimulate movement or motility.

11. A drug that has the opposite action of another drug or competes for the same receptor sites is an

_____ .

12. An ulcer in the stomach, duodenum, or other part of the GI system exposed to gastric juices is a

_____ .

Circle the BEST Answer

13. When giving a person an antacid, you do the following *except*
   A. ask about constipation or diarrhea
   B. observe for edema and signs and symptoms of heart failure
   C. observe for "coffee ground" vomitus and bloody or tarry stools
   D. observe for confusion

14. A person has an antacid and other drugs ordered. You give the other drugs
   A. 30 minutes before giving the antacid
   B. 1 hour before or 2 hours after giving the antacid
   C. 1 hour after giving the antacid
   D. with the antacid

15. A person had an order for a histamine blocker. You give the drug
   A. before meals
   B. with food or milk
   C. with an antacid
   D. on an empty stomach

16. Which statement about Cytotec is *false*?
   A. It is a gastro-intestinal prostaglandin.
   B. It is given on an empty stomach.
   C. Diarrhea may develop after 2 weeks of therapy.
   D. Its generic name is misoprostol.

17. Lansoprazole (Prevacid) is given
   A. daily for 6 to 8 days
   B. after breakfast
   C. before a meal
   D. at bedtime

18. Which statement about Carafate is *false*?
   A. Its generic name is sucralfate.
   B. It is given 1 hour before each meal and at bedtime.
   C. It is a coating agent.
   D. It is given after meals and at bedtime.

19. Metoclopramide (Reglan) is given
   A. 15 minutes before meals and at bedtime
   B. 30 minutes before meals and at bedtime
   C. 30 minutes after meals
   D. 60 minutes after meals

Fill in the Blanks

For questions 20-29 write out the meaning of each abbreviation.

20. g _____

_____

21. GERD _____

_____

22. GI _____

_____

23. MAR _____

_____

24. mcg _____

_____

25. mg _____

_____

26. mL _____

_____

27. NSAID _____

_____

28. PPI _____

_____

29. PUD _____

_____

30. The digestive system is also called the _____

_____.

31. The alimentary canal extends from the _____
_____ to the _____.

32. Digestion begins in the _____

_____.

33. Another term for mouth is _____

_____.

34. The _____ is a muscular tube that
extends from the pharynx to the stomach.

35. Involuntary muscle contractions that move food down
the esophagus through the alimentary canal is

_____.

36. GERD is commonly called _____,
_____ , and _____.

37. The goals of drug therapy for GERD and PUD are to

A. _____

B. _____

C. _____

Matching
Match the brand name of the histamine (H₂)-receptor antagonist with its generic name.

38. _____ Tagamet

39. _____ Pepcid

40. _____ Axid

41. _____ Zantac

A. famotidine
B. nizatidine
C. cimetidine
D. ranitidine

Match the brand name of the proton pump inhibitor with its generic name.

42. _____ Nexium

43. _____ Prevacid

44. _____ Prilosec

45. _____ Protonix

46. _____ Aciphex

A. lansoprazole
B. pantoprazole
C. esomeprazole
D. omeprazole
E. rabeprazole

Match the brand name of the anti-spasmodic agent with its generic name.

47. _____ Atropine Sulfate

48. _____ Bentyl

49. _____ Robinul

50. _____ Cantil

51. _____ Pamine

52. _____ Pro-Banthine

53. _____ Scopace

A. methscopolamine
B. atropine
C. mepenzolate
D. scopolamine
E. glycopyrrolate
F. dicyclomine
G. propantheline

True/False
Circle T if the statement is true. Circle F if the statement is false.

54. T   F   Some antacids are high in sodium.

55. T   F   A person taking an antacid has hypertension. You should measure his or her BP.

56. T   F   Histamine (H$_2$)-receptor antagonists are also called histamine blockers.

57. T   F   When giving a person a histamine blocker, you observe for confusion.

58. T   F   Prostaglandins inhibit gastric juice secretion and protect the stomach and duodenal lining from ulcers.

59. T   F   Proton pump inhibitors block gastric acid production.

60. T   F   Proton pump inhibitor tablets or capsules may be opened, crushed, or chewed.

61. T   F   A person taking metoclopramide (Reglan) may have restlessness, involuntary movements, and facial grimacing.

62. T   F   Anti-spasmodic agents result in increased gastric juices and increased GI motility.

63. T   F   When giving an anti-spasmodic drug, you measure blood pressure and the radial pulse.

Independent Learning Activities

- Obtain index cards. On each card, write the name of a drug class, observations to make when giving drugs in this class, and what to report and record. Here is an example:
  Drug Class: Antacids
  Observations:
  Report and record:
- Make flash cards for each of the drugs in the following tables. Include the generic name of the drug, the brand name, dose, action, clinical use, and comments.
  Commonly Used Antacids—Table 25-1
  Histamine (H$_2$)-Receptor Antagonists—Table 25-2
  Proton Pump Inhibitors—Table 25-3
  Anti-Spasmodic Agents—Table 25-4
- Ask your instructor to tell you which of the drugs in Tables 25-1 through 25-4 are used in your agency. For each drug, place a star on your drug card.

Fill in the Blanks: Key Terms

Use these terms to complete questions 1–12.

Anti-diarrheals   Emesis   Nausea
Anti-emetics   Fecal impaction Retching
Constipation   Griping   Vomiting
Diarrhea   Laxatives   Vomitus

1. Substances that cause evacuation of the bowel are
   _____.

2. The food and fluids expelled from the stomach
   through the mouth is _____.

3. _____ are drugs that relieve the
   symptoms of diarrhea.

4. Severe and spasm-like pain in the abdomen caused by
   an intestinal disorder is _____.

5. A _____ is the prolonged retention
   and build-up of feces in the rectum.

6. The involuntary, labored, spasmodic contractions of
   the abdominal and respiratory muscles without
   vomitus is called _____.

7. Another term for vomiting or vomitus is
   _____.

8. The passage of a hard, dry stool is _____.

9. Drugs used to treat nausea and vomiting are
   _____.

10. The sensation of abdominal discomfort that may lead
    to the urge or need to vomit is _____.

11. The frequent passage of liquid stools is _____.

12. _____ occurs when stomach contents
    are expelled through the mouth.

Circle the BEST Answer

13. Anti-emetics are more effective if given
    A. before the onset of nausea
    B. before bedtime
    C. after the onset of nausea
    D. after breakfast
14. A side effect of butyrophenones is
    A. nausea
    B. dizziness
    C. sedation
    D. constipation
15. Metoclopramide (Reglan) is useful in treating nausea
    and vomiting associated with
    A. over-eating
    B. pregnancy
    C. anesthesia
    D. GI cancers

16. Anti-cholinergic agents are used to relieve nausea and
    vomiting associated with
    A. mental illness
    B. motion sickness
    C. over-eating
    D. pain
17. Benzodiazepines reduce nausea and vomiting. They also
    A. control diarrhea
    B. reduce infections
    C. reduce anxiety associated with chemotherapy
    D. prevent constipation
18. Which drug class is used only for persons receiving
    chemotherapy?
    A. anti-cholinergic agents
    B. cortico-steroids
    C. cannabinoids
    D. laxatives
19. Aprepitant (Emend) is used with a cortico-steroid and a
    A. serotonin antagonist
    B. anti-cholinergic agent
    C. cannabinoids
    D. dopamine agent
20. A person is taking a stimulant laxative by mouth.
    This type of laxative acts within
    A. 1 to 2 hours
    B. 3 to 5 hours
    C. 6 to 10 hours
    D. 11 to 12 hours
21. Saline laxatives act by
    A. drawing water into the intestine
    B. lubricating the intestinal wall
    C. increasing bulk in the intestines
    D. irritating the intestines
22. Bulk-producing laxatives are given with a full glass of
    A. soda
    B. water
    C. milk
    D. sport drink
23. When giving a laxative you
    A. give small amounts of water
    B. follow directions on the MAR
    C. ignore patient complaints of abdominal discomfort
    D. give it with food
24. Systemic anti-diarrheal agents
    A. absorb excess water to cause a formed stool
    B. absorb irritants or bacteria causing the diarrhea
    C. reduce peristalsis and GI motility
    D. reduce flatus

Fill in the Blanks

For questions 25-32 write out the meaning of each abbreviation.

25. GI _____

    _____

26. h _____

    _____

27. MAR _____

    _____

28. mg _____

    _____

29. mL _____

    _____

30. MI _____

    _____

31. PO _____

    _____

32. VC _____

    _____

33. Retching is also called _____

    _____.

34. Lubricant laxatives and _____ are used to prevent constipation in persons who should not strain during defecation.

35. Fecal softeners are often called _____ and _____.

Matching

Match the brand name of the anti-diarrheal agent with its generic name.

36. _____ Motofen
37. _____ Lomotil
38. _____ Imodium
39. _____ Paregoric
40. _____ Lactinex
41. _____ Pepto-Bismol

A. opium
B. difenoxin with atropine
C. bismuth subsalicylate
D. loperamide
E. diphenoxylate with atropine
F. lactobacillus acidophilus

Match the brand name of the anti-emetic agent with its generic name.

42. _____ Thorazine
43. _____ Perphenazine
44. _____ Compazine
45. _____ Anzemet
46. _____ Tigan
47. _____ Kytril
48. _____ Zofran
49. _____ Dramamine
50. _____ Benadryl
51. _____ Atarax
52. _____ Antivert
53. _____ Decadron
54. _____ Ativan
55. _____ Emend

A. prochlorperazine
B. chlorpromazine
C. perphenazine
D. trimethobenzamide
E. granisetron
F. dolasetron
G. dimenhydrinate
H. ondansetron
I. dexamethasone
J. diphenhydramine
K. meclizine
L. hydroxyzine
M. lorazepam
N. aprepitant

True/False

Circle T if the statement is true. Circle F if the statement is false.

56. T F   High-fiber diets, fluids, and activity can prevent constipation.

57. T F   Liquid feces may seep from the anus of a person with a fecal impaction.

58. T   F   To prevent dehydration, fluid lost through diarrhea is replaced.

59. T   F   Older persons are at risk for dehydration from diarrhea.

60. T   F   Dopamine antagonists are used for nausea and vomiting.

61. T   F   Bulk-forming laxatives may be used to control certain types of diarrhea.

62. T   F   Stimulant and saline laxatives are routinely used as bowel preparations.

Independent Learning Activities

* Obtain index cards. On each card, write the name of a drug class, observations to make when giving drugs in this class, and what to report and record. Here is an example:
  Drug Class: Dopamine Agents
  Observations:
  Report and record:
* Make flash cards for each of the drugs in the following tables. Include the generic name of the drug, the brand name, dose, action, clinical use, and comments.
  Anti-Emetic Agents—Table 26-1
  Laxatives—Table 26-2
  Anti-Diarrheal Agents—Table 26-3
* Ask your instructor to tell you which of the drugs in Tables 26-1 through 26-3 are used in your agency. For each drug, place a star on your drug card.

27 Drugs Used to Treat Diabetes and Thyroid Diseases

Fill in the Blanks: Key Terms
Use these terms to complete questions 1–14.

Anti-thyroid agents
Anti-diabetic agents
Cretinism
Diabetes
Hyperglycemia

Hyperthyroidism
Hypoglycemia
Hypo-glycemic agents
Hypothyroidism
Insulin

Lactic acid
Lactic acidosis
Myxedema
Thyroid replacement hormones

1. A hormone produced by the pancreas is _____.

2. _____ is a disease that occurs from the excess production of thyroid hormones.

3. Another term for congenital hypothyroidism is
_____.

4. A build-up of lactic acid in the blood is _____.

5. _____ are drugs that lower the blood glucose level.

6. _____ is a disorder in which the body cannot produce or use insulin properly.

7. Drugs used to suppress the production of thyroid hormones are _____.

8. Hypothyroidism that occurs during adult life is called
_____.

9. Low sugar in the blood is _____.

10. _____ are drugs used to prevent or relieve the symptoms of diabetes.

11. Drugs that replace thyroid hormones in the treatment of hypothyroidism are _____.

12. A product of glucose metabolism is _____.

13. The disease that results from inadequate thyroid hormone production is _____.

14. High sugar in the blood is _____.

Circle the BEST Answer
15. Diabetes that develops during pregnancy is
    A. type 1
    B. type 2
    C. type 3
    D. gestational diabetes
16. Hypoglycemia is caused by
    A. too much insulin or diabetic drugs
    B. too little insulin or diabetic drugs
    C. eating too much food
    D. too little exercise
17. Goiter is an enlarged
    A. pancreas
    B. thyroid gland
    C. stomach
    D. intestines

18. After it is opened, an insulin bottle is discarded in
    A. 10 days
    B. 20 days
    C. 30 days
    D. 40 days
19. Which is *not* a sign or symptom of hypoglycemia?
    A. fatigue
    B. sweating
    C. dizziness
    D. flushed face
20. Which is *not* a sign or symptom of hyperglycemia?
    A. thirst
    B. dry mouth
    C. trembling
    D. frequent urination
21. The following statements are about metformin (Glucophage). Which statement is *false*?
    A. It increases the amount of glucose produced by the liver.
    B. It is used alone or with other oral anti-diabetic agents.
    C. The initial dose is 500 mg twice daily.
    D. Taking the drug with meals helps reduce side effects.
22. Which drug is *not* a second-generation sulfonylurea?
    A. glimepiride (Amaryl)
    B. glipizide (Glucotrol)
    C. chlorpropamide (Diabinese)
    D. glyburide (Glynase)
23. You are giving a person repaglinide (Prandin). You should give this drug
    A. 1 minute to 30 minutes before a meal
    B. 1 minute to 30 minutes after a meal
    C. 60 minutes before a meal
    D. 60 minutes after a meal
24. Precose and miglitol (Glyset) are given
    A. at the start of each main meal
    B. after each main meal
    C. 30 minutes before each main meal
    D. at bedtime

Fill in the Blanks
For questions 25-34 write out the meaning of each abbreviation.

25. F _____

_____

26. g _____

_____

27. GI _____

_____

28. mcg _____

_____

29. mg _____

_____

30. mL _____

_____

31. TSH _____

_____

32. T_3 _____

_____

33. T_4 _____

_____

34. TZD _____

_____

35. When giving an oral anti-diabetic or oral hypo-glycemic agent, you assist the nurse by

A. Measuring blood _____

B. Noting the person's _____ level

C. Noting when and what the person _____

36. When giving thyroid replacement hormones, you assist the nurse by

A. Measuring vital signs and using the _____ to measure heart rate

B. Asking about _____ elimination

C. Measuring _____

D. Observing for signs and symptoms of _____

Matching
Match the term with its definition.

37. _____ Onset

38. _____ Peak

39. _____ Duration

A. When the insulin will have the greatest effect
B. The length of time that the insulin is active in the body
C. The time required for the insulin to have an initial effect or action

Match the brand name of the sulfonylurea with its generic name.

40. _____ Diabinese

41. _____ Tolinase

42. _____ Orinase

43. _____ Amaryl

44. _____ Glucotrol

45. _____ Glucotrol XL

46. _____ Glynase

A. glimepiride
B. chlorpropamide
C. glyburide
D. tolazamide
E. glipizide
F. glipizide XL
G. tolbutamide

Match the brand name of the meglitinide agent with its generic name.

47. _____ Prandin

48. _____ Starlix

A. repaglinide
B. nateglinide

Match the brand name of the thiazolidinedione (TZD) agent with its generic name.

49. _____ Actos

50. _____ Avandia

A. rosiglitazone
B. pioglitazone

Match the brand name of the alpha-glucosidase inhibitor with its generic name.

51. _____ Precose

52. _____ Glyset

A. acarbose
B. miglitol

Match the brand name of the thyroid hormone with its generic name.

53. _____ Synthroid

54. _____ Cytomel

55. _____ Thyrolar

A. liothyronine
B. liotrix
C. levothyroxine

Match the brand name of the anti-thyroid drug with its generic name.

56. _____ Propacil

57. _____ Tapazole

A. methimazole
B. propylthiouracil

True/False
Circle T if the statement is true. Circle F if the statement is false.

58. T   F   Diabetes must be controlled to prevent complications.

59. T   F   For refrigerated insulin, the bottle is shaken to warm and re-mix it.

60. T   F   Signs and symptoms of hypoglycemia are more likely to occur when insulin reaches its peak.

61. T   F   A person is taking a sulfonylurea. Hypoglycemia is a possible side effect.

Independent Learning Activities
- Obtain index cards. On each card, write the name of a drug class, observations to make when giving drugs in this class, and what to report and record. Here is an example:
  Drug Class: Insulin
  Observations:
  Report and record:
- Make flash cards for each of the drugs in the following tables. Include the generic name of the drug, the brand name, dose, action, clinical use, and comments.
  Insulin—Table 27-2
  Sulfonylurea Oral Hypo-Glycemic Agents—Table 27-3
  Meglitinide Oral Hypo-Glycemic Agents—Table 27-4
  Thiazolidinedione Oral Hypo-Glycemic Agents—Table 27-5
  Thyroid Hormones—Table 27-6
- Ask your instructor to tell you which of the drugs in Tables 27-2 through 27-6 are used in your agency. For each drug, place a star on your drug card.
- Review your state regulations and your job description to see if you are permitted to give insulin by the subcutaneous route or by inhalation.

28 Cortico-Steroids and Gonadal Hormones

Fill in the Blanks: Key Terms
Use these terms to complete questions 1–11.

Androgens
Cortico-steroids
Endometriosis
Estrogen

Eunuchism
Gonads
Gluco-corticoids
Hypogonadism

Mineralo-corticoids
Progesterone
Testosterone

1. The female hormone is _____.

2. _____ is a condition in which the male lacks male hormones.

3. The hormone associated with body changes that favors implantation of the fertilized ovum, pregnancy, and lactation is _____.

4. The reproductive glands are called _____.

5. _____ are hormones that maintain fluid and electrolyte balance.

6. _____ is the male hormone.

7. A condition in which the tissue that lines the inside of the uterus grows outside the uterus is _____ _____.

8. Steroid hormones that produce masculine effects are _____.

9. Hormones that regulate carbohydrate, protein, and fat metabolism are _____.

10. _____ is a condition in which the body does not produce enough testosterone.

11. Hormones secreted by the adrenal cortex of the adrenal gland are _____.

Circle the BEST Answer
12. The generic name of Florinef is
    A. amcinonide
    B. fludrocortisone
    C. desonide
    D. prednisone
13. Florinef is used with gluco-corticoids to
    A. control blood pressure
    B. control nausea and vomiting
    C. treat acne
    D. prevent pregnancy
14. Cortico-steroid therapy may mask signs and symptoms of
    A. hypoglycemia
    B. hyperglycemia
    C. infection
    D. hypogonadism

15. The adult dose for mineralo-corticoids is
    A. 0.1 mg daily
    B. 1 mg daily
    C. .01 mg daily
    D. 1.1 mg daily
16. Gluco-corticoids are given
    A. before meals
    B. with meals
    C. after meals
    D. at bedtime
17. When giving estrogen and progestins, you measure vital signs and
    A. urine output
    B. color of nail beds
    C. weight
    D. observe for constipation
18. Progesterone and the progestins are used to treat the following *except*
    A. amenorrhea
    B. break-through uterine bleeding
    C. endometriosis
    D. hypertension

Fill in the Blanks
For questions 19–21 write out the meaning of each abbreviation.

19. g _____
    _____

20. mg _____
    _____

21. PO _____
    _____

22. When giving mineralo-corticoids and gluco-corticoids, you assist the nurse by

    A. Measuring vital _____

    B. Measuring _____

    C. Measuring intake and _____

    D. Observing for signs and symptoms of _____

    E. Observing level of alertness and orientation to person, time, and _____

    F. Testing stools for occult _____

Matching

Match the brand name of the estrogen with its generic name.

23. _____ Premarin

24. _____ Menest

25. _____ Estrace

26. _____ Ogen

A. estradiol
B. conjugated estrogen
C. estropipate
D. esterified estrogen

Match the brand name of the progestin with its generic name.

27. _____ Provera

28. _____ Aygestin

29. _____ Ovrette

30. _____ Progesterone

A. norethindrone
B. medroxyprogesterone
C. progesterone
D. norgestrel

Match the brand name of the androgen with its generic name.

31. _____ Striant

32. _____ Methitest

A. methyltestosterone
B. testosterone

True/False

Circle T if the statement is true. Circle F if the statement is false.

33. T   F   Gluco-corticoids are given for their anti-inflammatory and anti-allergenic effects.

34. T   F   Persons taking gluco-corticoids for at least 1 week may abruptly stop therapy.

35. T   F   Androgens may be used to treat breast cancer in post-menopausal women.

36. T   F   Androgens may cause hypoglycemia in persons with diabetes.

37. T   F   Androgens are given on an empty stomach.

Independent Learning Activities

- Obtain index cards. On each card, write the name of a drug class, observations to make when giving drugs in this class, and what to report and record. Here is an example:
  Drug Class: Mineralo-corticoids
  Observations:
  Report and record:
- Make flash cards for each of the drugs in the following tables. Include the generic name of the drug, the brand name, dose, action, clinical use, and comments.
  Estrogens—Table 28-2
  Progestins—Table 28-3
  Androgens—Table 28-4
- Ask your instructor to tell you which of the drugs in Tables 28-2 through 28-4 are used in your agency. For each drug, place a star on your drug card.

29 Drugs Used in Men's and Women's Health

Fill in the Blanks: Key Terms
Use these terms to complete questions 1–6.

Contraception   Impotence   Oral contraceptives
Erectile dysfunction   Leukorrhea   Priapism

1. Another term for birth control pills is _____
   _____ .

2. The process or method used to prevent pregnancy is
   _____ .

3. _____ is a prolonged or constant
   erection.

4. An abnormal whitish vaginal discharge is
   _____ .

5. The inability of the male to have an erection is
   _____ .

6. Another term for erectile dysfunction is
   _____ .

Circle the BEST Answer
7. Which drug is used to treat genital herpes?
   A. fluconazole oral tablets (Diflucan)
   B. metronidazole oral tablets (Flagyl)
   C. acyclovir oral tablets (Zovirax)
   D. doxycycline (Vibramycin)
8. The combination oral contraceptive pill contains
   A. estrogen only
   B. progestin only
   C. estrogen and progestin
   D. testosterone and estrogen
9. Combination pills are packaged with 28 tablets.
   The last 7 tablets contain
   A. iron
   B. estrogen
   C. progestin
   D. testosterone
10. Which statement about levonorgestrel/ethinyl estradiol
    (Seasonale) is *false*?
    A. It is a combination oral contraceptive.
    B. The woman has only 2 menstrual periods a year.
    C. The package has 84 active tablets.
    D. The package has 7 tablets that contain no hormones.
11. Which side effect from a contraceptive signals a
    serious complication?
    A. nausea
    B. vaginal bleeding
    C. dizziness
    D. weight gain
12. A transdermal contraceptive
    A. contains estrogen and progestin
    B. has no side effects
    C. is taken orally
    D. is taken daily

13. Alfuzosin (Uroxatral) and tamsulosin (Flomax) are
    used to treat
    A. genital infections
    B. mild leukorrhea
    C. mild to moderate urinary obstruction in men
       with BPH
    D. erectile dysfunction
14. Alfuzosin (Uroxatral) is given
    A. before the same meal each day
    B. immediately after the same meal each day
    C. 2 hours after a meal each day
    D. 1 hour before the same meal each day
15. Tamsulosin (Flomax) is given about
    A. 30 minutes before the same meal each day
    B. 30 minutes after the same meal each day
    C. 60 minutes before the same meal each day
    D. 60 minutes after the same meal each day
16. A person has dizziness and tachycardia 15 minutes after
    taking the first dose of tamsulosin (Flomax). You should
    A. call the doctor
    B. scold the person for taking the drug on an empty
       stomach
    C. have the person lie down and tell the nurse
    D. let the person walk alone in the hallway
17. Dutasteride (Avodart) and finasteride (Proscar) do the
    following *except*
    A. reduce BPH symptoms
    B. improve urine flow
    C. reduce the need for surgery
    D. control genital infections
18. Finasteride (Proscar) 5 mg is ordered for the person.
    In the drug drawer you find finasteride (Propecia)
    1 mg tablets. You
    A. call the pharmacist
    B. give 5 tablets of Propecia
    C. hold the dose and ask the nurse what to do
    D. talk with the pharmacy technician
19. A person taking sildenafil (Viagra) tells you he has
    problems seeing the color green. You
    A. tell him to reduce the dosage
    B. report and record the symptoms to the nurse
    C. call the physician
    D. ask him to stop joking with you

Fill in the Blanks
For questions 20–25 write out the meaning of each
abbreviation.

20. BPH _____

_____

21. ED _____

22. MAR _____

23. mg _____

24. STD _____

25. TURP _____

Matching
Match the brand name of the drug for genital infections with its generic name.

26. _____ Diflucan
27. _____ Flagyl
28. _____ Rocephin
29. _____ Tetracycline
30. _____ Zovirax
31. _____ Vibramycin

A. acyclovir
B. ceftriaxone
C. fluconazole
D. metronidazole
E. tetracycline
F. doxycycline

Match the brand name of the alpha-1 adrenergic blocking agent with its generic name.

32. _____ Uroxatral
33. _____ Flomax

A. tamsulosin
B. alfuzosin

Match the brand name of the anti-androgen agent with its generic name.

34. _____ Avodart
35. _____ Proscar

A. dutasteride
B. finasteride

Match the brand name of the drug used for erectile dysfunction with its generic name.

36. _____ Viagra
37. _____ Cialis
38. _____ Levitra

A. tadalafil
B. sildenafil
C. vardenafil

True/False
Circle T if the statement is true. Circle F if the statement is false.

39. T F When applying a transdermal contraceptive, you assist the nurse by measuring blood pressure in the supine and sitting positions.

40. T F A transdermal contraceptive patch is applied to skin that is irritated.

41. T F A transdermal contraceptive patch may be applied on a breast.

42. T F Alfuzosin (Uroxatral) tablets may be chewed or crushed.

43. T F Drugs used for erectile dysfunction are taken 30 minutes to 4 hours before sexual activity.

44. T F A person taking tadalafil (Cialis) develops angina. He should take his nitroglycerin.

45. T F Another term for benign prostatic hypertrophy is enlarged prostate.

Independent Learning Activities
• Obtain index cards. On each card, write the name of a drug class, observations to make when giving drugs in this class, and what to report and record. Here is an example:
Drug Class: Oral Contraceptives
Observations:
Report and record:

- Make flash cards for each of the drugs in the following tables. Include the generic name of the drug, the brand name, dose, action, clinical use, and comments.
  Drugs Used to Treat Genital Infections—Table 29-2
  Drugs Used in Obstetrics—Table 29-3
  Drugs Used for Erectile Dysfunction—Table 29-4
- Ask your instructor to tell you which of the drugs in Tables 29-2 through 29-4 are used in your agency. For each drug, place a star on your drug card.

30 Drugs Used to Treat Urinary System Disorders

Fill in the Blanks: Key Terms
Use these terms to complete questions 1–7.

Cystitis
Healthcare-associated
  infection

Over-active bladder
Prostatitis
Pyelonephritis

Urethritis
Urinary anti-microbial agents

1. Inflammation of the bladder is called _____
   _____.

2. _____ is inflammation of the prostate.

3. Substances that have an antiseptic effect on the urine
   and urinary tract are called _____.

4. An infection that develops in a person cared for in
   any setting where health care is given is a
   _____.

5. A term for inflammation of the urethra is
   _____.

6. A syndrome characterized by urinary frequency,
   urgency, and incontinence is an _____.

7. _____ is an inflammation of the
   kidney pelvis.

Circle the BEST Answer
8. Fosfomycin (Monurol) granules are dissolved in
   A. 60 mL water
   B. 60 mL hot water
   C. 90 to 120 mL hot water
   D. 90 to 120 mL water
9. When giving a quinolone antibiotic, you do the
   following *except*
   A. measure height and weight
   B. note the amount and color of urine
   C. ask about urgency, burning, or other problems
   D. ask about vision problem
10. A person taking a quinolone antibiotic has hematuria.
    He or she should drink
    A. 1 to 3 glasses of water daily
    B. 4 to 5 glasses of water daily
    C. 6 to 7 glasses of water daily
    D. 8 to 12 glasses of water daily

11. Nalidixic acid (NegGram) is taken
    A. on an empty stomach
    B. before meals
    C. with meals
    D. anytime

Fill in the Blanks
**For questions 12–18 write out the meaning of each
abbreviation.**

12. g _____
    _____

13. GI _____
    _____

14. HAI _____
    _____

15. mg _____
    _____

16. mL _____
    _____

17. OAB _____
    _____

18. UTI _____
    _____

Matching
Match the brand name of the quinolone antibiotic with its generic name.

19. _____ NegGram

20. _____ Noroxin

A. norfloxacin
B. nalidixic acid

Match the brand name of the anti-bacterial agent with its generic name.

21. _____ Mandelamine

22. _____ Macrodantin and Furadantin

A. methenamine mandelate
B. nitrofurantoin

Match the brand name of the anti-cholinergic drug with its generic name.

23. _____ Enablex

24. _____ Ditropan

25. _____ Vesicare

26. _____ Detrol

27. _____ Sanctura

A. oxybutynin
B. darifenacin
C. solifenacin
D. trospium
E. tolterodine

True/False
Circle T if the statement is true. Circle F if the statement is false.

28. T F   Women and older persons are at high risk for UTIs.

29. T F   Fosfomycin (Monurol) is used as a single dose to treat uncomplicated acute cystitis in women.

30. T F   Fosfomycin (Monurol) may be taken with or without food.

31. T F   A person taking a quinolone antibiotic may have visual problems during the first few days.

32. T F   Photo-sensitivity is a side effect of quinolone antibiotics.

33. T F   Methenamine mandelate (Mandelamine) should be taken with meals and at bedtime.

34. T F   Methenamine mandelate (Mandelamine) tablets may be crushed.

35. T F   Nitrofurantoin (Macrodantin, Furadantin) is given with food or milk.

36. T F   Numbness and tingling in the extremities are side effects of nitrofurantoin (Macrodantin, Furadantin).

37. T F   Anti-cholinergic drugs also are known as urinary anti-spasmodic agents.

38. T F   A person is taking an anti-cholinergic drug for an OAB. Possible side effects are dry mouth, blurred vision, constipation, confusion, and sedation.

Independent Learning Activities
- Obtain index cards. On each card, write the name of a drug class, observations to make when giving drugs in this class, and what to report and record. Here is an example:
  Drug Class: Fosfomycin antibiotics
  Observations:
  Report and record:
- Make flash cards for each of the drugs in the following tables. Include the generic name of the drug, the brand name, dose, action, clinical use, and comments.
  Quinolone Urinary Antibiotics—Table 30-1
  Urinary Anti-Cholinergic Agents—Table 30-2
- Ask your instructor to tell you which of the drugs in Tables 30-1 and 30-2 are used in your agency. For each drug, place a star on the drug card.

Drugs Used to Treat Eye Disorders

Fill in the Blanks: Key Terms
Use these terms to complete questions 1–3.

Miosis   Mydriasis   Osmotic agents

1. A term for dilation of the pupil is _____.

2. Drugs that cause fluid to be drawn from outside of the vascular system into the blood are _____ _____.

3. _____ is the narrowing of the pupil.

Circle the BEST Answer

4. Two different eye drops are ordered for a person at the same time. You give the first drug. How long should you wait before giving the second drug?
   A. 1 minute
   B. 5 minutes
   C. 10 minutes
   D. 15 minutes

5. You are giving a person a carbonic anhydrase inhibitor. Which statement is *false*?
   A. It reduces intra-ocular pressure.
   B. It may be given to a person who is allergic to sulfonamide antibiotics.
   C. Oral dose forms are given with food or milk.
   D. Contact lenses are removed for topical dose forms.

6. Which statement about echothiophate iodine (Phospholine Iodide) is *false*?
   A. It causes miosis (pupil constriction).
   B. You assist the nurse by taking vital signs.
   C. It decreases IOP.
   D. It has no side effects.

7. A person taking a beta-adrenergic blocking agent has bradycardia and hypotension. You
   A. tell the nurse
   B. record the symptoms in the chart
   C. tell the nurse and record the symptoms in the chart
   D. call the doctor

8. Which statement about natamycin (Natacyn) is *false*?
   A. Its generic name is natamycin.
   B. It is used to treat fungal infections of the eye.
   C. It may cause sensitivity to bright light.
   D. It has no side effects.

9. Trifluridine (Viroptic) is used to treat
   A. fungal infections of the eye
   B. herpes infections of the eye
   C. intra-ocular pressure
   D. cataracts

10. Ophthalmic antibiotics are used to treat
    A. fungal infections of the eye
    B. herpes infections of the eye
    C. intra-ocular pressure
    D. superficial eye infections

11. Cortico-steroids are used for
    A. allergic reactions of the eye
    B. fungal infections of the eye
    C. herpes infections of the eye
    D. intra-ocular pressure

12. Flurbiprofen (Ocufen) is
    A. a cholinergic agent
    B. an anti-inflammatory agent
    C. an anti-cholinergic agent
    D. a prostaglandin agonist

13. Cromolyn (Crolom) is
    A. a cholinergic agent
    B. an anti-allergic agent
    C. an anti-cholinergic agent
    D. a prostaglandin agonist

Fill in the Blanks
For questions 14-20 write out the meaning of each abbreviation.

14. g _____
    _____

15. GI _____
    _____

16. IOP _____
    _____

17. kg _____
    _____

18. mg _____
    _____

19. mL _____
    _____

20. PO _____
    _____

21. Cholinergic agents lower IOP in persons with glaucoma. They also reverse pupil _____ after eye surgery or eye exams.

22. Adrenergic agents cause pupil dilation and _____ to bright light.

23. Anti-cholinergic agents dilate pupils and may cause _____ to bright light.

Matching

Match the brand name of the osmotic agent with its generic name.

24. _____ Osmoglyn
25. _____ Ismotic

A. isosorbide
B. glycerin

Match the brand name of the carbonic anhydrase inhibitor with its generic name.

26. _____ Diamox
27. _____ Azopt
28. _____ Trusopt

A. brinzolamide
B. dorzolamide
C. acetazolamide

Match the brand name of the cholinergic agent with its generic name.

29. _____ Isopto-Carbachol
30. _____ Isopto-Carpine

A. pilocarpine
B. carbachol

Match the brand name of the adrenergic agent with its generic name.

31. _____ Iopidine
32. _____ Alphagan P
33. _____ Propine
34. _____ Vasoclear
35. _____ Prefrin
36. _____ Murine Plus

A. dipivefrin hydrochloride
B. tetrahydrozoline hydrochloride
C. apraclonidine
D. phenylephrine
E. brimonidine
F. naphazoline hydrochloride

Match the brand name of the beta-adrenergic blocking agent with its generic name.

37. _____ Betoptic
38. _____ Ocupress
39. _____ Betagan
40. _____ OptiPranolol
41. _____ Timoptic

A. betaxolol hydrochloride
B. timolol maleate
C. metipranolol
D. carteolol
E. levobunolol hydrochloride

Match the brand name of the prostaglandin agonist with its generic name.

42. _____ Lumigan
43. _____ Xalatan
44. _____ Travatan

A. travoprost
B. latanoprost
C. bimatoprost

Match the brand name of the anti-cholinergic agent with its generic name.

45. _____ Isopto-Atropine
46. _____ Cyclogyl
47. _____ Isopto-Homatropine
48. _____ Isopto-Hyoscine
49. _____ Mydriacyl

A. homatropine hydrobromide
B. scopolamine hydrobromide
C. atropine sulfate
D. cyclopentolate hydrochloride
E. tropicamide

Match the brand name of the cortico-steroid with its generic name.

50. _____ Decadron
51. _____ FML
52. _____ Lotemax
53. _____ HMS
54. _____ Econopred Plus
55. _____ Vexol

A. medrysone
B. dexamethasone
C. rimexolone
D. prednisolone
E. loteprednol
F. fluorometholone

Match the brand name of the ophthalmic anti-inflammatory agent with its generic name.

56. _____ Ocufen

57. _____ Profenal

58. _____ Voltaren

59. _____ Acular

A. flurbiprofen
B. suprofen
C. diclofenac
D. ketorolac

Match the brand name of the ophthalmic antihistamine with its generic name.

60. _____ Optivar

61. _____ Emadine

62. _____ Elestat

63. _____ Zaditor

64. _____ Patanol

A. ketotifen
B. olopatadine
C. azelastine
D. emedastine
E. epinastine

Match the brand name of the anti-allergic agent with its generic name.

65. _____ Crolom

66. _____ Alomide

67. _____ Alamast

68. _____ Alocril

A. nedocromil
B. lodoxamide
C. cromolyn
D. pemirolast

True/False
Circle T if the statement is true. Circle F if the statement is false.

69. T   F   A cataract results in damage to the optic nerve.

70. T   F   Glaucoma is a clouding of the lens in the eye.

71. T   F   Eye drops should be applied before eye ointments.

72. T   F   You applied an eye ointment to a person. You should wait a few hours to apply his or her eye drops.

73. T   F   Osmotic agents used to treat glaucoma reduce intra-ocular pressure.

74. T   F   Glycerin (Osmoglyn) and isosorbide (Ismotic) are oral osmotic agents.

75. T   F   A person taking a cholinergic agent or a cholinesterase inhibitor may have problems adjusting to changes in light.

76. T   F   Prostaglandin agonists may gradually change a person's eye color.

77. T   F   Prolonged or frequent use of topical ophthalmic antibiotics should be avoided.

78. T   F   Ketorolac (Acular) is used to relieve eye itching from seasonal allergies.

79. T   F   Antihistamines are used to relieve the signs and symptoms associated with allergic conjunctivitis.

80. T   F   Artificial tear solutions lubricate dry eyes.

Independent Learning Activities
- Obtain index cards. On each card, write the name of a drug class, observations to make when giving drugs in this class, and what to report and record. Here is an example:
Drug Class: Osmotic agents
Observations:
Report and record:

32 Drugs Used in the Treatment of Cancer

Fill in the Blanks: Key Terms
Use these terms to complete questions 1–7.

Alopecia   Cancer   Metastasis   Tumor
Benign tumor   Malignant tumor   Stomatitis

1. The spread of cancer to other body parts is _____
   _____ .

2. A tumor that does not spread to other body parts is a
   _____ .

3. _____ is inflammation of the mouth.

4. Another term for hair loss is _____ .

5. A _____ is a new growth of abnormal
   cells.

6. Another term for a malignant tumor is _____
   _____ .

7. A tumor that invades and destroys nearby tissue and
   can spread to other body parts is a _____ .

Circle the BEST Answer
8. A person has had surgery for cancer. After surgery
   you expect that the person will
   A. need pain-relief drugs
   B. have skin breakdown
   C. want many visitors
   D. have hair loss

9. Side effects from chemotherapy may include all the
   following *except*
   A. alopecia
   B. stomatitis
   C. burns to the skin
   D. bleeding and infection

10. A risk factor for cancer is
    A. not smoking tobacco
    B. limiting time in the sun
    C. high-fat diet
    D. regular exercise

11. Which of the following is *not* a sign or symptom of
    cancer?
    A. an obvious change in an existing mole
    B. a sore that heals
    C. changes in bowel or bladder habits
    D. unusual bleeding or discharge

True/False
Circle T if the statement is true. Circle F if the statement is false.

12. T F Malignant tumors may be life-threatening.

13. T F Benign tumors spread to other body parts.

14. T F Cancer occurs in all age groups.

15. T F Sun, sunlamps, and tanning booths can lead to skin cancer.

16. T F Radiation therapy can destroy both cancer cells and normal cells.

17. T F Hormone therapy may be used to treat certain types of cancer.

Independent Learning Activities
• Review your state regulations and your job description to see if you are allowed to give oral dose forms of drugs used
  to treat cancer.
• If you are permitted to give oral dose forms of drugs used to treat cancer, ask your instructor which drugs in Table 32-1 you
  are permitted to give. Write the drug, usual dose, toxicity, and major indicators on an index card.

33 Drugs Affecting Muscles and Joints

Fill in the Blanks: Key Terms
Use these terms to complete questions 1–3.

Clonus   Hyper-reflexia   Spasm

1. Increased reflex actions are called _____.

2. Rapidly alternating involuntary contraction and relaxation of skeletal muscles are called _____.

3. An involuntary muscle contraction of sudden onset is a _____.

Circle the BEST Answer

4. You can control
   A. voluntary muscles
   B. involuntary muscles
   C. cardiac muscle
   D. smooth muscle

5. Centrally acting skeletal muscle relaxants are used to
   A. relieve cardiac spasm
   B. relieve acute muscle spasm
   C. relieve acute muscle spasm
   D. relieve gout pain

6. All centrally acting skeletal muscle relaxants cause some degree of
   A. anxiety
   B. depression
   C. hyperactivity
   D. sedation

7. When giving centrally acting skeletal muscle relaxants, you assist the nurse by measuring vital signs and
   A. urine output
   B. weight
   C. observing level of alertness
   D. fluid intake

8. Which statement about dantrolene (Dantrium) is *false*?
   A. It decreases muscle spasm, clonus, and hyper-reflexia.
   B. Its generic name is dantrolene.
   C. The person may experience photo-sensitivity, diarrhea, and drowsiness.
   D. It is used for persons with a stroke.

9. Baclofen (Lioresal) is given to persons with
   A. gout
   B. arthritis
   C. multiple sclerosis and spinal cord injuries
   D. cerebral palsy

10. Allopurinol (Aloprim) is given
    A. with food or milk
    B. before meals
    C. after meals
    D. on an empty stomach

11. A person taking allopurinol (Zyloprim) develops itching and a rash. You
    A. give the drug as ordered
    B. only give next dose if approved by the nurse
    C. ask the person if he wants to take the drug
    D. call the pharmacist

12. Probenecid is given
    A. with food or milk
    B. before meals
    C. after meals
    D. on an empty stomach

Fill in the Blanks
For questions 13–17 write out the meaning of each abbreviation.

13. CNS _____

    _____

14. g _____

    _____

15. GI _____

    _____

16. mg _____

    _____

17. PO _____

    _____

Matching
Match the brand name of the centrally acting skeletal muscle relaxant with its generic name.

18. _____ Soma

19. _____ Flexeril

20. _____ Skelaxin

21. _____ Robaxin

22. _____ Norflex

23. _____ Zanaflex

A. cyclobenzaprine
B. carisoprodol
C. tizanidine
D. methocarbamol
E. metaxalone
F. orphenadrine citrate

True/False
Circle T if the statement is true. Circle F if the statement is false.

24. T   F   Centrally acting skeletal muscle relaxants depress the central nervous system.

25. T   F   The generic name for Lioresal is baclofen.

26. T   F   Non-steroidal anti-inflammatory agents and cortico-steroids are used to treat gout.

27. T   F   The brand names for allopurinol are Aloprim and Zyloprim.

28. T   F   Colchicine is used to relieve joint pain caused by an acute gout attack.

29. T   F   When taking colchicine, the person should drink 8 to 12 glasses of fluid daily.

30. T   F   When taking probenecid, the person should drink 8 to 12 glasses of fluid daily.

Independent Learning Activities
- Obtain index cards. On each card, write the name of a drug class, observations to make when giving drugs in this class, and what to report and record. Here is an example:
  Drug Class: Centrally Acting Skeletal Muscle Relaxants
  Observations:
  Report and record:
- Make flash cards for each of the drugs in the following table. Include the generic name of the drug, the brand name, dose, action, clinical use, and comments.
  Centrally Acting Muscle Relaxants—Table 33-1
- Ask your instructor to tell you which of the drugs in Table 33-1 are used in your agency. For each drug, place a star on your drug card.

34 Drugs Used to Treat Infections

Fill in the Blanks: Key Terms
Use these terms to complete questions 1–19.

Aerobe
Anaerobe
Antibiotics
Anti-microbial agents
Bacteria

Carrier
Fungi
Germs
Healthcare-associated
   infection

Infection
Microbe
Microorganism
Non-pathogen
Normal flora

Opportunistic infection
Pathogen
Protozoa
Secondary infection
Viruses

1. Plants that live on other plants or animals are called
   _____.

2. A disease state resulting from the invasion and growth of microbes in the body is an _____.

3. _____ are microbes that live and grow in a certain area.

4. A _____ is a microbe that is harmful and can cause an infection.

5. _____ are microbes that grow in living cells.

6. A microbe that lives and grows in the presence of oxygen is called an _____.

7. An _____ is a microbe that lives and grows in the absence of oxygen.

8. A microbe that does not usually cause an infection is a
   _____.

9. An infection caused by non-pathogens in a person with a weakened immune system is an _____.

10. An infection caused by a microbe that follows the first infection caused by a different microbe is a _____.

11. A _____ is an infection that develops in a person cared for in any setting where health care is given.

12. Anti-microbials derived from living micro-organisms are called _____.

13. A human or animal that is a reservoir for microbes but does not have the signs and symptoms of infection is a _____.

14. A small living plant or animal seen only with a microscope is a _____.

15. One-celled animals that can infect the blood, brain, intestines, and other body areas are _____.

16. _____ are one-celled plant life that multiply rapidly and can cause an infection in any body system.

17. Chemicals that eliminate pathogens are _____.

18. Bacteria is another term for _____.

19. Another term for microorganism is _____.

Circle the BEST Answer
20. Which system protects the body from disease and infection?
    A. immune
    B. gastrointestinal
    C. respiratory
    D. endocrine

21. Anti-bacterial agents destroy
    A. fungus
    B. viruses
    C. bacteria
    D. protozoa

22. Before giving an anti-microbial drug, you always
    A. put on gloves
    B. check for allergies
    C. take vital signs
    D. check the person's blood glucose

23. A person is started on an anti-microbial drug. You should observe him or her for at least the first
    A. 5 to 10 minutes after the drug is given
    B. 15 to 20 minutes after the drug is given
    C. 20 to 30 minutes after the drug is given
    D. 40 to 60 minutes after the drug is given

24. A person is having a serious allergic reaction after the first dose of an anti-microbial drug. He or she may have the following *except*
    A. hives
    B. bleeding
    C. wheezing
    D. dyspnea

25. Neomycin (Neo-fradin) can cause
    A. hearing loss
    B. loss of sight
    C. loss of taste
    D. loss of touch

26. A person is taking a cephalo-sporin. You should report and record the following *except*
    A. diarrhea
    B. thrush
    C. bleeding and easy bruising
    D. normal vital signs

27. A common side effect of penicillin is
    A. blurred vision
    B. discolored teeth
    C. hearing loss
    D. diarrhea
28. A side effect of a quinolone antibiotic is photo-sensitivity. A person taking this drug should do the following *except*
    A. avoid exposure to sunlight, sunlamps, and tanning beds
    B. apply a sunscreen when outdoors
    C. stay indoors
    D. wear long-sleeved garments, a hat, and sunglasses when outdoors
29. Ciprofloxacin (Cipro) is taken
    A. with meals
    B. before meals
    C. on an empty stomach
    D. 2 hours after meals
30. Which drug class may stain teeth if given during tooth development?
    A. ketolides
    B. tetracyclines
    C. penicillins
    D. macrolides
31. A woman who is nursing her child is started on a tetracycline. She should
    A. continue to nurse her infant
    B. nurse the infant only once a day
    C. feed the infant formula or cow's milk
    D. nurse the infant 2 hours after taking the drug
32. Ethambutol (Myambutol) is given
    A. before breakfast
    B. with food or milk
    C. on an empty stomach
    D. at bedtime
33. Isoniazid (INH) is given
    A. 30 minutes after eating
    B. with food or milk
    C. on an empty stomach
    D. with juice
34. Which anti-tubercular drug may cause reddish-orange secretions?
    A. ethambutol (Myambutol)
    B. isoniazid (INH)
    C. rifampin (Rifadin)
    D. clindamycin (Cleocin)
35. A person taking metronidazole (Flagyl) should avoid
    A. milk and milk products
    B. alcoholic beverages and products containing alcohol
    C. fruit juices
    D. vegetable juices
36. Which drug can cause hearing damage?
    A. clindamycin (Cleocin)
    B. metronidazole (Flagyl)
    C. tinidazole (Tindamax)
    D vancomycin (Vancocin)
37. Flucytosine (Ancobon) is given
    A. twice a day
    B. three times a day
    C. every 6 hours
    D. every 12 hours

38. Griseofulvin (Fulvicin and Grifulvin) are used to treat
    A. ringworm of the scalp, body, nails, and feet
    B. fungal infections affecting the mouth and pharynx
    C. fungal infections affecting the heart and lungs
    D. fungal infections affecting the blood and urinary tract
39. A person is taking ketoconazole (Nizoral). Which statement is *false*?
    A. The drug is taken at least 2 hours before drugs that reduce stomach acidity.
    B. The drug is taken with food.
    C. The person should avoid alcoholic beverages and products containing alcohol.
    D. The drug is taken on an empty stomach.
40. A possible side effect of acyclovir (Zovirax) is hypotension. You should do the following *except*
    A. measure blood pressure in the supine and standing positions
    B. provide for safety
    C. remind the person to rise slowly from a supine or sitting position
    D. have the person stand if he or she feels faint
41. Atazanavir (Reyataz) is given
    A. once daily with food
    B. once daily on an empty stomach
    C. 2 hours after eating
    D. before breakfast
42. You should mix didanosine (Videx) powder with
    A. fruit juice
    B. four ounces of water
    C. milk
    D. liquids containing acid
43. Women who are or may become pregnant should *not* take
    A. emtricitabine (Emtriva)
    B. atazanavir (Reyataz)
    C. didanosine (Videx)
    D. efavirenz (Sustiva)
44. Oseltamivir (Tamiflu) is given
    A. with food or milk
    B. once daily on an empty stomach
    C. 2 hours after eating
    D. before breakfast
45. A person taking zanamivir (Relenza) has shortness of breath and chest soreness. He or she must
    A. skip a dose
    B. continue to take the drug
    C. stop taking the drug and seek medical attention
    D. stop taking the drug

Fill in the Blanks
For questions 46-60 write out the meaning of each abbreviation.

46. AIDS _____

    _____

47. CDC _____

    _____

48. g _____

    _____

49. GI _____

50. HAI _____

51. HBV _____

52. HIV _____

53. IM _____

54. IV _____

55. kg _____

56. mg _____

57. mL _____

58. STD _____

59. TB _____

60. UTI _____

61. A _____ infection is in a body part.

62. A _____ infection involves the whole body.

63. You should report signs and symptoms of infection to the nurse _____.

64. When applying a topical anti-fungal agent, you should wear _____.

65. A person using a topical anti-fungal agent has redness, swelling, blistering, or oozing at the sight. These may signal an _____.

66. Another term for herpes zoster is _____.

Matching
Match the term with its definition.

67. _____ Antibodies
68. _____ Antigens
69. _____ Phagocytes
70. _____ Lymphocytes
71. _____ B lymphocytes (B cells)
72. _____ T lymphocytes (T cells)

A. Abnormal or unwanted substances that cause the body to produce antibodies
B. Cells that destroy invading cells
C. White blood cells that produce antibodies
D. Normal body substances that recognize abnormal or unwanted substances
E. Cells that cause the production of antibodies that circulate in the plasma
F. White blood cells that digest and destroy microbes and other unwanted substances

Match the brand name of the cephalo-sporin with its generic name.

73. _____ Ceclor
74. _____ Duricef
75. _____ Omnicef
76. _____ Suprax
77. _____ Vantin
78. _____ Cefzil
79. _____ Cedax
80. _____ Zinacef
81. _____ Keflex
82. _____ Velosef

A. cefuroxime
B. cefdinir
C. ceftibuten
D. cefaclor
E. cephalexin
F. cefadroxil
G. cefixime
H. cefpodoxime
I. cefprozil
J. cephradine

Match the brand name of the macrolide with its generic name.

83. _____ Zithromax

84. _____ Biaxin

85. _____ Eryc

A. clarithromycin
B. erythromycin
C. azithromycin

Match the brand name of the penicillin with its generic name.

86. _____ Amoxil

87. _____ Principen

88. _____ Geocillin

89. _____ Dicloxacillin

90. _____ Oxacillin

91. _____ Penicillin VK

A. oxacillin
B. amoxicillin
C. carbenicillin
D. penicillin V potassium
E. dicloxacillin
F. ampicillin

Match the brand name of the quinolone with its generic name.

92. _____ Cipro

93. _____ Factive

94. _____ Levaquin

95. _____ Maxaquin

96. _____ Avelox

97. _____ NegGram

98. _____ Noroxin

99. _____ Floxin

A. ofloxacin
B. ciprofloxacin
C. norfloxacin
D. gemifloxacin
E. nalidixic acid
F. levofloxacin
G. moxifloxacin
H. lomefloxacin

Match the brand name of the sulfonamide with its generic name.

100. _____ Sulfadiazine

101. _____ Azulfidine

102. _____ Gantrisin

103. _____ Bactrim

104. _____ Pediazole

A. co-trimoxazole
B. sulfasalazine
C. sulfadiazine
D. erythromycin-sulfisoxazole
E. sulfisoxazole

Match the brand name of the tetracycline with its generic name.

105. _____ Declomycin

106. _____ Vibramycin

107. _____ Minocin

108. _____ Sumycin

A. minocycline
B. demeclocycline
C. tetracycline
D. doxycycline

Match the brand name of the anti-tubercular drug with its generic name.

109. _____ Myambutol

110. _____ INH

111. _____ Rifadin

A. ethambutol
B. rifampin
C. isoniazid

Match the brand name of the antibiotic with its generic name.

112. _____ Cleocin

113. _____ Flagyl

114. _____ Tindamax

115. _____ Vancocin

A. clindamycin
B. vancomycin
C. tinidazole
D. metronidazole

Match the brand name of the systemic anti-fungal agent with its generic name.

116. _____ Diflucan

117. _____ Ancobon

118. _____ Fulvicin

119. _____ Sporanox

120. _____ Nizoral

121. _____ Lamisil

A. ketoconazole
B. itraconazole
C. fluconazole
D. terbinafine
E. griseofulvin
F. flucytosine

Match the brand name of the anti-viral agent with its generic name.

122. _____ Zovirax

123. _____ Famvir

124. _____ Valtrex

125. _____ Ziagen

126. _____ Reyataz

127. _____ Videx

128. _____ Sustiva

129. _____ Emtriva

130. _____ Epiver and Epivir-HBV

131. _____ Zerit and Zerit XR

132. _____ Retrovir

133. _____ Symmetrel

134. _____ Tamiflu

135. _____ Relenza

136. _____ Virazole and Rebetol

A. valacyclovir
B. atazanavir
C. efavirenz
D. famciclovir
E. didanosine
F. abacavir
G. acyclovir
H. emtricitabine
I. stavudine
J. amantadine hydrochloride
K. zanamivir
L. ribavirin
M. oseltamivir
N. zidovudine
O. lamivudine

True/False

Circle T if the statement is true. Circle F if the statement is false.

137. T F Microbes are everywhere.

138. T F When a non-pathogen is transmitted from its natural site to another site or host, it becomes a pathogen.

139. T F Immunity means that a person has protection against a disease or condition.

140. T F An infection can become life-threatening before an older person has obvious signs and symptoms.

141. T F The goal of anti-microbial therapy is to eliminate the infection.

142. T F Anti-microbials are usually given at regular intervals to maintain blood levels of the drug.

143. T F Diarrhea, nausea, vomiting, and abnormal taste are the most common side effects of macrolides.

144. T F A person taking a sulfonamide should drink water several times a day.

145. T F Tetracyclines are given 1 hour before or 2 hours after the person ingests antacids or milk.

146. T F Isoniazid (INH) is used to prevent and treat TB.

147. T F You should refrigerate clindamycin (Cleocin) suspension.

148. T F Itraconazole (Sporanox) is given with a full meal.

149. T F All drug forms of didanosine (Videx) are given on an empty stomach.

150. T F Inhaled broncho-dilators should be taken before zanamivir (Relenza) is inhaled.

Independent Learning Activities

- Obtain index cards. On each card, write the name of a drug class, observations to make when giving drugs in this class, and what to report and record. Here is an example:

  Drug Class: Amino-Glycosides

  Observations:

  Report and record:

- Make flash cards for each of the drugs in the following tables. Include the generic name of the drug, the brand name, dose, action, clinical use, and comments.

  Cephalo-sporins—Table 34-1

  Macrolides—Table 34-2

  Penicillins—Table 34-3

  Quinolones—Table 34-4

  Sulfonamides—Table 34-5

  Tetracyclines—Table 34-6

  Topical Anti-Fungal Agents—Table 34-7

- Ask your instructor to tell you which of the drugs in Tables 34-1 through 34-7 are used in your agency. For each drug, place a star on your drug card.

35 Nutrition and Herbal and Dietary Supplement Therapy

Fill in the Blanks: Key Terms
Use these terms to complete questions 1–15.

Aspiration
Calorie
Enteral nutrition
Gastrostomy tube
Jejunostomy
Malnutrition

Naso-gastric (NG) tube
Naso-duodenal tube
Naso-intestinal tube
Naso-jejunal tube
Nutrient
Nutrition

Parenteral nutrition
Percutaneous endoscopic gastrostomy
 (PEG) tube
Regurgitation

1. A substance that is ingested, digested, absorbed, and used by the body is a _____.

2. Any disorder of nutrition is _____.

3. A _____ is the amount of energy produced when the body burns food.

4. The processes involved in the ingestion, digestion, absorption, and use of foods and fluids by the body is called _____.

5. Breathing fluid, food, vomitus, or an object into the lungs is _____.

6. Giving nutrients into the gastro-intestinal tract through a feeding tube is _____.

7. Giving nutrients through a catheter inserted into a vein is _____.

8. A _____ is inserted through a surgically created opening in the stomach.

9. A feeding tube inserted into a surgically created opening in the jejunum of the small intestine is a _____.

10. A feeding tube inserted through the nose into the stomach is a _____.

11. A feeding tube inserted through the nose into the duodenum of the small intestine is a _____.

12. A _____ is a feeding tube inserted through the nose into the small intestine.

13. A feeding tube inserted through the nose into the jejunum of the small intestine is a _____.

14. A feeding tube inserted into the stomach through a small incision made through the skin is a _____.

15. The backward flow of stomach contents into the mouth is _____.

Circle the BEST Answer
16. Vitamin K is needed for
    A. healthy hair, skin, and mucous membranes
    B. muscle tone
    C. healthy eyes
    D. blood clotting

17. Thiamin is
    A. vitamin B_1
    B. vitamin B_2
    C. vitamin B_3
    D. vitamin B_{12}

18. Ascorbic acid is
    A. vitamin A
    B. vitamin C
    C. vitamin D
    D. vitamin E

19. The major function of iron is
    A. growth and metabolism
    B. fluid balance
    C. nerve function
    D. it allows red blood cells to carry oxygen

20. Which is an oral nutritional supplement?
    A. Echinacea
    B. Ginseng
    C. Ensure
    D. Niacin

21. A continuous tube feeding is given
    A. every 2 hours
    B. every 4 hours
    C. every 6 hours
    D. over a 24-hour period

22. A person is on TPN. You may
    A. increase the flow rate
    B. hang a new bag
    C. observe the person closely
    D. decrease the flow rate

Fill in the Blanks
For questions 23-33 write out the meaning of each abbreviation.

23. AIDS _____
_____

24. BPH _____
_____

25. CNS _____
_____

26. GI _____
_____

27. IV _____
   _____

28. MAR _____
   _____

29. mg _____
   _____

30. mL _____
   _____

31. NG _____
   _____

32. PEG _____
   _____

33. TPN _____
   _____

34. Protein is needed for _____ and _____.

35. Carbohydrates provide _____ and _____ for bowel elimination.

36. Fats provide _____, add _____ to food, and help the body use certain _____.

37. The body stores vitamins _____, _____, _____ and _____.

38. Vitamin _____ and the _____ complex vitamins must be ingested daily.

39. Minerals are needed for _____ and _____ formation, nerve and muscle function, fluid balance, and other body processes.

40. Water is ingested through _____ and _____.

True/False
Circle T if the statement is true. Circle F if the statement is false.

41. T F Good nutrition is needed for growth, healing, and body functions.

42. T F Nutrients include fats, proteins, carbohydrates, vitamins, minerals, and water.

43. T F Fats, proteins, and carbohydrates give the body fuel for energy.

44. T F Persons who are malnourished are at risk for infections and organ failure.

45. T F Parenteral nutrition is often called hyperalimentation.

46. T F You may insert a feeding tube or check its placement.

47. T F A person is receiving a tube feeding. To prevent regurgitation and aspiration maintain Fowler's or semi-Fowler's position after the feeding.

48. T F The health benefit claims made for herbal and dietary supplements have been proven.

Independent Learning Activities
• Review your state regulations to see if you are allowed to give tube feedings. Also check to see if the procedure is in your job description.

Review of Textbook Appendix A

Fill in the Blanks

Roman Numerals

Express the following in Arabic numerals.

1. ii _____
2. iv _____
3. v _____
4. viii _____
5. x _____
6. xv _____
7. ix _____
8. xix _____
9. i _____
10. iii _____
11. vi _____
12. vii _____
13. xi _____
14. L _____
15. C _____
16. D _____
17. M _____

Express the following in Roman numerals.

18. 3 _____
19. 6 _____
20. 17 _____
21. 20 _____

Fractions

22. The numerator of $\frac{1}{5}$ is _____
23. The denominator of $\frac{3}{8}$ is _____
24. The smaller the denominator number, the _____ the portion is.
25. The larger the denominator number, the _____ the portion is.

Identify which fraction is larger.

26. $\frac{1}{4}$ or $\frac{1}{2}$ _____
27. $\frac{1}{8}$ or $\frac{1}{4}$ _____

28. $\frac{1}{2}$ or $\frac{3}{4}$ _____
29. $\frac{1}{3}$ or $\frac{2}{3}$ _____

Identify whether the fraction is proper or improper.

30. $\frac{3}{5}$ _____
31. $\frac{1}{4}$ _____
32. $\frac{7}{4}$ _____
33. $\frac{3}{2}$ _____

Reduce the fraction to its lowest terms.

34. $\frac{3}{6}$ _____
35. $\frac{1}{12}$ _____
36. $\frac{4}{16}$ _____
37. $\frac{5}{25}$ _____

Add these fractions. Reduce each sum to its lowest terms.

38. $\frac{1}{4} + \frac{3}{4} =$ _____
39. $\frac{1}{5} + \frac{2}{5} =$ _____
40. $\frac{1}{8} + \frac{5}{8} =$ _____
41. $\frac{1}{7} + \frac{4}{7} =$ _____
42. $\frac{1}{6} + \frac{2}{6} =$ _____
43. $1 \frac{1}{2} + 2 \frac{1}{2} =$ _____
44. $2 \frac{1}{3} + 4 \frac{2}{3} =$ _____

Multiply the following.

45. 2.75 x 0.5 = _____
46. 4.5 x 1.25 = _____

Change the decimal fraction to a common fraction.

47. 0.3 = _____
48. 0.5 = _____
49. 0.7 = _____
50. 0.25 = _____
51. 0.33 = _____
52. 0.66 = _____
53. 0.75 = _____

Change the common fraction to a decimal fraction.

54. ½ = _____

55. ²/₃ = _____

56. ¾ = _____

57. ⁵/₆ = _____

58. ⁷/₈ = _____

Percents

Change the percent to a common fraction.

59. 10% = _____

60. 25% = _____

61. 50% = _____

62. 75% = _____

63. 100% = _____

64. 33% = _____

65. 125% = _____

Change the percent to a decimal fraction.

66. 10% = _____

67. 25% = _____

68. 50% = _____

69. 75% = _____

70. 33% = _____

71. 125% = _____

Systems of Weights and Measures

Express the common household equivalent for each of the following.

72. 1 quart = _____ cups

73. 1 pint = _____ cups

74. 1 cup = _____ ounces

75. 1 tablespoon = _____ teaspoons

76. 1 teaspoon = _____ mL

Express the following common metric equivalents.

77. 1000 milliliter (mL) = _____ L

78. 1000 milligrams (mg) = _____ g

79. 1000 micrograms (mcg) = _____ mg

80. 1,000,000 micrograms (mcg) = _____ g

81. 1000 grams (g) = _____ kg

Convert the following milligrams to grams.

82. 0.5 mg = _____ g

83. 250 mg = _____ g

84. 500 mg = _____ g

Convert the following grams to milligrams.

85. 0.75 g = _____ mg

86. 0.3 g = _____ mg

Conversion Problems

87. You have drug tablets that are 0.1 mg. You need to give 0.4 mg. How many tablets will you give?

_____

88. You have drug tablets that are 0.5 mg. You need to give 0.25 mg. What will you give?

_____

89. The doctor orders 150 mg of a drug. You have 100 mg tablets. How many tablets should you administer?

_____

90. The doctor orders 3 g of a drug. The drug label states the strength on hand is 0.5 g. How many tablets should you give?

_____

91. The doctor orders 0.75 mg of a drug. The drug label states the strength on hand is 0.25 mg. How many tablets should you give?

_____

92. The doctor orders 0.25 mg of a drug. The drug label states the strength on hand is 0.50 mg. How many tablets should you give?

_____

93. The doctor orders Lasix 40 mg. You have tablets that are 20 mg each. How many tablets will you give?

_____

94. The doctor orders digoxin 0.125 mg. You have tablets that are 0.25 mg. How many tablets will you give?

_____

95. The doctor orders Tylenol 300 mg. You have tablets that are 300 mg. How many tablets will you give?

_____

96. The doctor orders 500 mg of Cipro suspension. You have 250 mg/5 mL. How much will you give?

_____

97. The doctor orders Coumadin 15 mg PO. You have
10 mg tablets. How many tablets will you give?

_____

98. A person takes Aldomet 500 mg tablets twice a day.
How many total milligrams does the person take
in a day?

_____

99. The doctor orders Motrin 800 mg PO. You have
Motrin 400 mg. How many tablets will you give?

_____

Taking a Temperature

Name: _____   Date: _____

Quality of Life	S	U	Comments

Remembered to:
- Knock before entering the person's room.
- Address the person by name.
- Introduce yourself by name and title.
- Explain the procedure to the person before beginning and during the procedure.
- Protect the person's rights during the procedure.
- Handle the person gently during the procedure.

Pre-Procedure

1. Followed *Delegation Guidelines: Taking Temperatures.* Viewed *Promoting Safety and Comfort:*
   A. *Glass Thermometers*
   B. *Taking Temperatures*
2. For an oral temperature, asked the person not to eat, drink, smoke, or chew gum for at least 15 to 20 minutes or as required by agency policy.
3. Practiced hand hygiene.
4. Collected the following:
   A. Appropriate thermometer
   B. Probe and probe covers (if needed)
   C. Tissues
   D. Plastic covers if used (glass thermometers)
   E. Gloves
   F. Toilet tissue (rectal temperature)
   G. Water-soluble lubricant (rectal temperature)
   H. Towel (axillary temperature)
5. Plugged the oral or rectal probe into the electronic thermometer.
6. Decontaminated your hands.
7. Identified the person. Checked the ID bracelet against the assignment sheet. Called the person by name.
8. Provided for privacy.

Procedure

9. Positioned the person for an oral, rectal, axillary, or tympanic membrane temperature.
10. Put on gloves if contact with blood, body fluids.
11. Inserted the probe into a probe cover.
12. For a *glass thermometer:*
    A. Rinsed it in cold water if it was soaking in a disinfectant. Dried it with tissues.
    B. Checked it for breaks, cracks, or chips.
    C. Shook it below the lowest number. Held it by the stem.
    D. Inserted it into a plastic cover if used.

Date of Satisfactory Completion _____   Instructor's Initials _____

Procedure—cont'd	S	U	Comments

13. For an *oral temperature:*
  A. Asked the person to moisten his or her lips.
  B. Placed the covered probe at the base of the tongue and to one side. If a glass thermometer was used, placed the bulb end under the tongue and to one side.
  C. Asked the person to close the lips around the thermometer to hold it in place.
  D. Asked the person not to talk. Reminded the person not to bite down on a glass thermometer.
  E. Left a glass thermometer in place for 2 to 3 minutes or as required by agency policy.

14. For a *rectal temperature:*
  A. Put a small amount of lubricant on a tissue.
  B. Lubricated the bulb end of the thermometer.
  C. Exposed the anal area.
  D. Raised the upper buttock to expose the anus.
  E. Inserted the glass thermometer 1 inch into the rectum. Inserted an electronic thermometer ½ inch into the rectum. Did not force the thermometer.
  F. Held a glass thermometer in place for 2 minutes or as required by agency policy.

15. For an *axillary temperature:*
  A. Helped the person remove an arm from the gown. Did not expose the person.
  B. Dried the axilla with a towel.
  C. Placed the covered probe in the axilla. For a glass thermometer, placed the bulb end of the thermometer in the center of the axilla.
  D. Asked the person to place the arm over the chest to hold the thermometer in place. Held it and the arm in place if the person could not help.
  E. Left a glass thermometer in place for 5 to 10 minutes or as required by agency policy.

16. For a *tympanic membrane temperature:*
  A. Asked the person to turn his or her head so the ear was in front of you.
  B. Pulled up and back on the ear.
  C. Inserted the covered probe gently.

17. For an *electronic or tympanic membrane thermometer:*
  A. Started the thermometer.
  B. Held the probe in place until hearing a tone or seeing a flashing or steady light.
  C. Read the temperature on the display.
  D. Removed the probe. Pressed the eject button to discard the cover.

18. For a *glass thermometer:*
  A. Removed the glass thermometer.
  B. Used tissues to remove the plastic cover. Discarded the cover and tissues. Wiped the thermometer from the stem to the bulb with a tissue if no cover was used. Discarded the tissue.
  C. Read the thermometer.

19. Noted the person's name, temperature, and temperature site on the notepad or assignment sheet.
20. Returned the probe to the holder.

Date of Satisfactory Completion _____ Instructor's Initials _____

Procedure—cont'd	S	U	Comments
21. For a *rectal temperature:*			
A. Placed used toilet tissue on several thicknesses of toilet tissue.	___	___	_____
B. Placed the glass thermometer on clean toilet tissue.	___	___	_____
C. Wiped the anal area to remove excess lubricant and any feces.	___	___	_____
D. Covered the person.	___	___	_____
22. For an *axillary temperature:* Helped the person put the gown back on.	___	___	_____
23. Shook down the glass thermometer.	___	___	_____
24. Cleaned the glass thermometer according to agency policy. Returned it to the holder.	___	___	_____
25. Discarded tissues. Disposed of toilet tissue.	___	___	_____
26. Removed gloves. Decontaminated hands.	___	___	_____

Post-Procedure

	S	U	Comments
27. Provided for comfort.	___	___	_____
28. Placed the signal light within reach.	___	___	_____
29. Unscreened the person.	___	___	_____
30. Completed a safety check of the room.	___	___	_____
31. Returned the electronic or tympanic membrane thermometer to the charging unit.	___	___	_____
32. Decontaminated your hands.	___	___	_____
33. Reported and recorded the temperature. Noted the temperature site when reporting and recording. Reported any abnormal temperature at once.	___	___	_____

Date of Satisfactory Completion _____ Instructor's Initials _____

Taking a Pulse

Name: _____   Date: _____

	S	U	Comments

Quality of Life
Remembered to:
- Knock before entering the person's room.
- Address the person by name.
- Introduce yourself by name and title.
- Explain the procedure to the person before beginning and during the procedure.
- Protect the person's rights during the procedure.
- Handle the person gently during the procedure.

Pre-Procedure
1. Followed *Delegation Guidelines: Taking a Pulse.* Viewed *Promoting Safety and Comfort: Taking a Pulse.*
2. Asked a nursing team member to help you take an apical-radial pulse.
3. Practiced hand hygiene.
4. Collected a stethoscope and antiseptic wipes for an apical pulse or an apical-radial pulse.
5. Decontaminated your hands.
6. Identified the person. Checked the ID bracelet against the assignment sheet. Called the person by name.
7. Provided for privacy.

Procedure
8. Cleaned the earpieces and diaphragm with wipes.
9. Had the person sit or lie down.
10. For a *radial pulse:*
    A. Located the radial pulse. Used your first two or three middle fingers.
    B. Noted if the pulse was strong or weak, and regular or irregular.
    C. Counted the pulse for 30 seconds. Multiplied the number of beats by 2. Or counted the pulse for 1 minute if directed by the nurse and care plan, agency policy, or the pulse was irregular.
11. For an *apical pulse:*
    A. Exposed the nipple area of the left chest. Did not expose a woman's breasts.
    B. Warmed the diaphragm in your palm.
    C. Placed the earpieces in your ears.
    D. Found the apical pulse. Placed the diaphragm 2 to 3 inches to the left of the breastbone and below the left nipple.
    E. Counted the pulse for 1 minute. Noted if it was regular or irregular.
    F. Covered the person. Removed the earpieces.
12. For an *apical-radial pulse*:
    A. Followed steps 11 A-C.
    B. Found the apical pulse while your helper found the radial pulse.
    C. Gave the signal to begin counting.
    D. Counted the pulse for 1 minute.
    E. Gave the signal to stop counting.
    F. Subtracted the radial pulse from the apical pulse for the pulse deficit. Noted whether the pulse was regular or irregular.

Date of Satisfactory Completion _____   Instructor's Initials _____

Procedure—cont'd   S   U   Comments

13. Noted the person's name and pulse on the notepad
    or assignment sheet. For an apical-radial pulse, noted
    the apical and radial pulse rates and the pulse deficit.
    Noted the strength of the pulse. Noted if it was regular
    or irregular.

Post-Procedure

14. Provided for comfort.
15. Placed the signal light within reach.
16. Unscreened the person.
17. Completed a safety check of the room.
18. Cleaned the earpieces and diaphragm with the wipes.
19. Returned the stethoscope to its proper place.
20. Decontaminated your hands.
21. Reported and recorded your observations. Recorded the
    pulse rate and noted the site. Reported an abnormal
    pulse rate at once. For an apical-radial pulse, noted:
    A. The apical and radial pulse rates
    B. The pulse deficit

Date of Satisfactory Completion _____ Instructor's Initials _____

Counting Respirations

Name: _____   Date: _____

	S	U	Comments
Quality of Life			
Remembered to:			
• Knock before entering the person's room.	____	____	_____
• Address the person by name.	____	____	_____
• Introduce yourself by name and title.	____	____	_____
• Explain the procedure to the person before beginning and during the procedure.	____	____	_____
• Protect the person's rights during the procedure.	____	____	_____
• Handle the person gently during the procedure.	____	____	_____

Procedure

	S	U	Comments
1. Followed *Delegation Guidelines: Respirations*.	____	____	_____
2. Kept your fingers or stethoscope over the pulse site.	____	____	_____
3. Did not tell the person you are counting respirations.	____	____	_____
4. Began counting when the chest rises. Counted each rise and fall of the chest as 1 respiration.	____	____	_____
5. Noted the following:			
A. If respirations were regular	____	____	_____
B. If both sides of the chest rose equally	____	____	_____
C. The depth of respirations	____	____	_____
D. If the person had any pain or difficulty breathing	____	____	_____
E. An abnormal respiratory pattern	____	____	_____
6. Counted respirations for 30 seconds. Multiplied the number by 2. Counted respirations for 1 minute if directed by the nurse and care plan, if required by agency policy, or if respirations were abnormal or irregular.	____	____	_____
7. Noted the person's name, respiratory rate, and other observations on your notepad or assignment sheet.	____	____	_____

Post-Procedure

	S	U	Comments
8. Provided for comfort.	____	____	_____
9. Placed the signal light within reach.	____	____	_____
10. Unscreened the person.	____	____	_____
11. Completed a safety check of the room.	____	____	_____
12. Decontaminated your hands.	____	____	_____
13. Reported and recorded the respiratory rate and your observations. Reported abnormal respirations at once.	____	____	_____

Date of Satisfactory Completion _____   Instructor's Initials _____

Measuring Blood Pressure

Name: _____   Date: _____

Quality of Life	S	U	Comments

Remembered to:
- Knock before entering the person's room.
- Address the person by name.
- Introduce yourself by name and title.
- Explain the procedure to the person before beginning and during the procedure.
- Protect the person's rights during the procedure.
- Handle the person gently during the procedure.

Pre-Procedure
1. Followed *Delegation Guidelines: Blood Pressure.* Viewed *Promoting Safety and Comfort: Taking a Pulse and Blood Pressure.*
2. Practiced hand hygiene.
3. Collected the following:
   A. Sphygmomanometer
   B. Stethoscope
   C. Antiseptic wipes
4. Decontaminated your hands.
5. Identified the person. Checked the ID bracelet against the assignment sheet. Called the person by name.
6. Provided for privacy.

Procedure
7. Wiped the stethoscope earpieces and diaphragm with the wipes. Warmed the diaphragm in your palm.
8. Had the person sit or lie down.
9. Positioned the person's arm level with the heart. The palm was up.
10. Stood no more than 3 feet away from the manometer.
11. Exposed the upper arm.
12. Squeezed the cuff to expel any remaining air. Closed the valve on the bulb.
13. Found the brachial artery at the inner aspect of the elbow.
14. Placed the arrow on the cuff over the brachial artery. Wrapped the cuff around the upper arm at least 1 inch above the elbow. It was even and snug.
15. *One-step method:*
    A. Placed the stethoscope earpieces in your ears.
    B. Found the radial or brachial artery.
    C. Inflated the cuff until you could no longer feel the pulse. Noted this point.
    D. Inflated the cuff 30 mm Hg beyond the point where you last felt the pulse.
16. *Two-step method:*
    A. Found the radial or brachial artery.
    B. Inflated the cuff until you could no longer feel the pulse. Noted this point.
    C. Inflated the cuff 30 mm Hg beyond the point where you last felt the pulse.
    D. Deflated the cuff slowly. Noted the point when you felt the pulse.
    E. Waited 30 seconds.
    F. Placed the stethoscope earpieces in your ears.
    G. Inflated the cuff 30 mm Hg beyond the point where you felt the pulse return.

Date of Satisfactory Completion _____   Instructor's Initials _____

Procedure—cont'd

	S	U	Comments
17. Placed the diaphragm of the stethoscope over the brachial artery. Did not place it under the cuff.	___	___	_____
18. Deflated the cuff at an even rate of 2 to 4 millimeters per second. Turned the valve counter-clockwise to deflate the cuff.	___	___	_____
19. Noted the point where you heard the first sound. This is the systolic reading. It is near the point where the radial pulse disappeared.	___	___	_____
20. Continued to deflate the cuff. Noted the point where the sound disappeared. This is the diastolic reading.	___	___	_____
21. Deflated the cuff completely. Removed it from the person's arm. Removed the stethoscope earpieces from your ears.	___	___	_____
22. Noted the person's name and blood pressure on your notepad or assignment sheet.	___	___	_____
23. Returned the cuff to the case or wall holder.	___	___	_____

Post-Procedure

	S	U	Comments
24. Provided for comfort.	___	___	_____
25. Placed the signal light within reach.	___	___	_____
26. Unscreened the person.	___	___	_____
27. Completed a safety check of the room.	___	___	_____
28. Cleaned the earpieces and diaphragm with the wipes.	___	___	_____
29. Returned the equipment to its proper place.	___	___	_____
30. Decontaminated your hands.	___	___	_____
31. Reported and recorded the blood pressure. Reported an abnormal blood pressure at once.	___	___	_____

Date of Satisfactory Completion _____   Instructor's Initials _____

Measuring Weight and Height

Name: _____   Date: _____

Quality of Life	S	U	Comments

Remembered to:
- Knock before entering the person's room.
- Address the person by name.
- Introduce yourself by name and title.
- Explain the procedure to the person before beginning and during the procedure.
- Protect the person's rights during the procedure.
- Handle the person gently during the procedure.

Pre-Procedure
1. Followed *Delegation Guidelines: Measuring Weight and Height*. Viewed *Promoting Safety and Comfort: Measuring Weight and Height*.
2. Asked the person to void.
3. Practiced hand hygiene.
4. Brought the scale and paper towels to the person's room.
5. Decontaminated your hands.
6. Identified the person. Checked the ID bracelet against the assignment sheet. Called the person by name.
7. Provided for privacy.

Procedure
8. Placed the paper towels on the scale platform.
9. Raised the height rod.
10. Moved the weights to zero.
11. Had the person remove the robe and footwear. Assisted as needed.
12. Helped the person stand on the scale. The person stood in the center of the scale. Arms were at the person's sides.
13. Moved the weights until the balance pointer was in the middle.
14. Noted the weight on your notepad or assignment sheet.
15. Asked the person to stand very straight.
16. Lowered the height rod until it rests on the person's head.
17. Noted the height on your notepad or assignment sheet.
18. Raised the height rod. Helped the person step off of the scale.
19. Helped the person put on a robe and non-skid footwear if he or she would be up. Or helped the person back to bed.
20. Lowered the height rod. Adjusted the weights to zero if this is your agency's policy.

Post-Procedure
21. Provided for comfort.
22. Placed the signal light within reach.
23. Raised or lowered bed rails. Followed the care plan.
24. Unscreened the person.
25. Completed a safety check of the room.
26. Discarded the paper towels.
27. Returned the scale to its proper place.
28. Decontaminated your hands.
29. Reported and recorded the measurements.

Date of Satisfactory Completion _____   Instructor's Initials _____

Measuring Blood Glucose

Name: _____   Date: _____

Quality of Life	S	U	Comments

Remembered to:
- Knock before entering the person's room.
- Address the person by name.
- Introduce yourself by name and title.
- Explain the procedure to the person before beginning and during the procedure.
- Protect the person's rights during the procedure.
- Handle the person gently during the procedure.

Pre-Procedure
1. Followed *Delegation Guidelines: Blood Glucose Testing.* Viewed *Promoting Safety and Comfort: Blood Glucose Testing.*
2. Practiced hand hygiene.
3. Collected the following:
   A. Sterile lancet
   B. Anti-septic wipes
   C. Gloves
   D. Cotton balls
   E. Glucose meter
   F. Reagent strips—Used the correct ones for the meter. Checked the expiration date.
   G. Paper towels
   H. Washcloth
   I. Soap, towel, and wash basin
4. Read the manufacturer's instructions for the lancet and glucose meter.
5. Arranged your work area.
6. Identified the person. Checked the ID bracelet against the assignment sheet. Called the person by name.
7. Provided for privacy.
8. Raised the bed for body mechanics. The far bed rail was up if used.

Procedure
9. Helped the person to a comfortable position.
10. Assisted with hand washing.
11. Put on the gloves.
12. Prepared the supplies:
    A. Opened the anti-septic wipes.
    B. Removed a reagent strip from the bottle. Placed it on the paper towel. Placed the cap securely on the bottle.
    C. Prepared the lancet.
    D. Turned on the glucose meter.
13. Performed a skin puncture to obtain a drop of blood:
    A. Inspected the person's fingers. Selected a skin puncture site.
    B. Warmed the finger. Rubbed it gently or applied a warm washcloth.
    C. Massaged the hand and finger toward the puncture site.
    D. Lowered the finger below the person's waist.
    E. Held the finger with your thumb and forefinger. Used your non-dominant hand. Held the finger until step 13 K.

Date of Satisfactory Completion _____   Instructor's Initials _____

	S	U	Comments
Procedure—cont'd			
F. Cleaned the site with anti-septic wipe. Did not touch the site after cleaning.	____	____	_____
G. Let the site dry.	____	____	_____
H. Picked up the sterile lancet.	____	____	_____
I. Placed the lancet against the side of the finger or the top of the finger tip.	____	____	_____
J. Pushed the button on the lancet to puncture the skin.	____	____	_____
K. Wiped away the first blood drop. Used a cotton ball.	____	____	_____
L. Applied gentle pressure below the puncture site.	____	____	_____
M. Let a large drop of blood form.	____	____	_____
14. Collected and tested the specimen. Followed the manufacturer's instructions and agency procedures for the glucose meter used.			
A. Held the test area of the reagent strip close to the drop of blood.	____	____	_____
B. Lightly touched the reagent strip to the blood drop. Did not smear the blood.	____	____	_____
C. Set the timer on the glucose meter.	____	____	_____
D. Waited the length of time required by the manufacturer.	____	____	_____
E. Applied pressure to the puncture site until bleeding stopped. Used a cotton ball. If able, let the person apply pressure to the site.	____	____	_____
F. Read the result on the display. Noted the result and told the person the result.	____	____	_____
G. Turned off the glucose meter.	____	____	_____
15. Discarded the lancet into the sharps container.	____	____	_____
16. Discarded the cotton balls following agency policy.	____	____	_____
17. Removed and discarded the gloves. Decontaminated your hands.	____	____	_____
Post-Procedure			
18. Provided for comfort.	____	____	_____
19. Placed the signal light within reach.	____	____	_____
20. Lowered the bed to its lowest position.	____	____	_____
21. Raised or lowered bed rails. Followed the care plan.	____	____	_____
22. Unscreened the person.	____	____	_____
23. Discarded used supplies. Cleaned and returned the bath basin to its proper place.	____	____	_____
24. Completed a safety check of the room.	____	____	_____
25. Followed agency policy for soiled linen.	____	____	_____
26. Decontaminated your hands.	____	____	_____
27. Returned the glucose meter to its proper place.	____	____	_____
28. Reported and recorded the test results and your observations.	____	____	_____

Date of Satisfactory Completion _____   Instructor's Initials _____

Hand Washing

Name: _____   Date: _____

Quality of Life	S	U	Comments
Remembered to:			
• Knock before entering the person's room.	___	___	_____
• Address the person by name.	___	___	_____
• Introduce yourself by name and title.	___	___	_____

Procedure

	S	U	Comments
1. See *Promoting Safety and Comfort: Hand Hygiene*.			
2. Made sure you had soap, paper towels, an orange stick or nail file, and a wastebasket. Collected missing items.	___	___	_____
3. Pushed your watch up your arm 4 to 5 inches. Also pushed up uniform sleeves.	___	___	_____
4. Stood away from the sink. Made sure clothes did not touch the sink. Stood so the soap and faucet were easy to reach.	___	___	_____
5. Turned on and adjusted the water until it felt warm.	___	___	_____
6. Wet your wrists and hands. Kept your hands lower than your elbows.	___	___	_____
7. Applied about 1 teaspoon of soap to your hands.	___	___	_____
8. Rubbed your palms together and interlaced your fingers. Worked up a good lather. Performed this step for at least 15 seconds.	___	___	_____
9. Washed each hand and wrist thoroughly. Cleaned well between the fingers.	___	___	_____
10. Cleaned under the fingernails. Rubbed your fingertips against your palms.	___	___	_____
11. Cleaned under the fingernails with a nail file or orange stick if first hand washing of the day or hands were highly soiled.	___	___	_____
12. Rinsed wrists and hands well. Water flowed from the arms to the hands.	___	___	_____
13. Repeated steps 7-13 if needed.	___	___	_____
14. Dried your wrists and hands with paper towels. Patted dry, starting at your fingertips.	___	___	_____
15. Discarded the paper towel into the wastebasket.	___	___	_____
16. Turned off the faucets with clean, dry paper towels. Used a clean paper towel for each faucet.	___	___	_____
17. Discarded the paper towels into the wastebasket.	___	___	_____

Date of Satisfactory Completion _____   Instructor's Initials _____

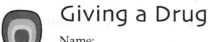
Giving a Drug

Name: _____   Date: _____

Quality of Life	S	U	Comments

Remembered to:
- Knock before entering the person's room.
- Address the person by name.
- Introduce yourself by name and title.
- Explain the procedure to the person before beginning and during the procedure.
- Protect the person's rights during the procedure.
- Handle the person gently during the procedure.

Pre-Procedure
1. Checked the drug order. (First safety check.) Focused on the right drug, right time, right dose, right person, right route.
2. Checked with the nurse if you had any questions.
3. Practiced hand hygiene.
4. Collected needed items (medication cup, juice, or a straw)
5. Unlocked the drug cart.
6. Read the order on the MAR.
7. Selected the right drug from the person's drawer.
8. Compared the drug order on the MAR against the pharmacy label on the drug container. (Second safety check.) Checked for the right drug, right time, right dose, right person, right route.
9. Checked the drug container for an expiration date.
10. Compared the drug order on the MAR against the pharmacy label on the drug container. (Third safety check.) Checked for the right drug, right time, right dose, right person, right route.
11. Opened the container. Poured the correct dosage from bottle. Returned extra drugs to the container. Did not open a unit dose container until at the person's bedside.
12. Closed the container. Compared the drug order on the MAR against the pharmacy label on the drug container. (Fourth safety check.) Checked for the right drug, right time, right dose, right person, right route.
13. Returned the container to the drawer.
14. Repeated steps 6-13 for each drug ordered for the person.
15. Locked the drug cart if left outside the person's room.

Procedure
16. Identified the person. Checked the ID bracelet against the MAR. Used at least two identifiers according to agency policy. Also called the person by name. Followed agency policy if using a bar code scanner.
17. Provided for privacy.
18. Obtained required measurements as noted on the MAR.
19. Positioned the person appropriately for the drug form.
20. Gave the person the drugs.

Post-Procedure
21. Discarded the medicine cup or unit dose packages.
22. Provided for the person's comfort.
23. Unscreened the person.
24. Completed a safety check before leaving the room.

Date of Satisfactory Completion _____   Instructor's Initials _____

Procedure—cont'd

	S	U	Comments
25. Practiced hand hygiene.	___	___	_____
26. Recorded the right documentation on the MAR:			
A. The date, time, drug name, dosage, and route of administration.	___	___	_____
B. The application site	___	___	_____
C. Name or initials	___	___	_____
27. Reported and recorded any specific patient or resident observations or concerns.	___	___	_____

Date of Satisfactory Completion _____   Instructor's Initials _____

Giving an Oral Drug—Solid Form

Name: _____   Date: _____

Quality of Life	S	U	Comments

Remembered to:
- Knock before entering the person's room.
- Address the person by name.
- Introduce yourself by name and title.
- Explain the procedure to the person before beginning and during the procedure.
- Protect the person's rights during the procedure.
- Handle the person gently during the procedure.

Pre-Procedure
1. Followed *Delegation Guidelines: Giving Oral Drugs*. Viewed *Promoting Safety and Comfort: Giving Oral Drugs*.
2. Checked the drug order. (First safety check.) Focused on the right drug, right time, right dose, right person, and right route.
3. Checked with the nurse if you had any questions.
4. Practiced hand hygiene.
5. Collected the following:
   A. MAR
   B. Water glass and water or other ordered liquid
   C. Straws
   D. Souffle cups
6. Unlocked the drug cart.
7. Read the order on the MAR.
8. Selected the right drug from the person's drawer or bin.
9. Compared the drug order on the MAR against the pharmacy label on the drug container. (Second safety check.) Checked for the right drug, right time, right dose, right person, right route.
10. Checked the drug container for an expiration date.
11. Compared the drug order on the MAR against the pharmacy label on the drug container. (Third safety check.) Checked for the right drug, right time, right dose, right person, right route.
12. Prepared the drug:
   A. Opened the container. Did not open a unit dose package until at the person's bedside.
   B. Poured the ordered dosage into the container cap or lid. Gently tapped on the container. Did not let the container touch the cap or lid.
   C. Returned extra tablets or capsules back into the container. Did not let the cap or lid touch the container.
   D. Poured the tablet or capsule from the lid into the souffle cup.
13. Closed the container. Compared the drug order on the MAR against the pharmacy label on the drug container. (Fourth safety check.) Checked for the right drug, right time, right dose, right person, right route.
14. Returned the container to the drawer or bin.
15. Repeated steps 7-14 for each drug ordered for the person.
16. Locked the drug cart if you left it outside the person's room.

Date of Satisfactory Completion _____   Instructor's Initials _____

Procedure

17. Identified the person. Checked the ID bracelet against the MAR. Used at least two identifiers according to agency policy. Called the person by name. Followed agency policy if using a bar code scanner.   _____ _____   _____
18. Provided for privacy.   _____ _____   _____
19. Obtained required measurements as noted on the MAR. Noted the measurement on the MAR.   _____ _____   _____
20. Positioned the person in a sitting or Fowler's position. Or positioned the person as directed by the nurse, care plan, and MAR.   _____ _____   _____
21. Let the person drink a small amount of water. Provided a straw if the person preferred.   _____ _____   _____
22. Gave the person the drugs. If a unit dose system was used:
    A. Handed the drug package to the person. Asked him or her to read the label.   _____ _____   _____
    B. Asked the person to hand the package back to you.   _____ _____   _____
    C. Opened the package.   _____ _____   _____
    D. Placed the contents into the person's hand.   _____ _____   _____
23. Gave the person a full glass of water or ordered fluid. Provided a straw if the person preferred. Encouraged the person to drink all of the water or other fluid.   _____ _____   _____
24. Stayed with the person to make sure he or she swallowed all of the drugs. If necessary, checked the person's mouth—under the tongue and between teeth and the cheeks.   _____ _____   _____

Post-Procedure

25. Discarded the souffle cup or unit dose packages.   _____ _____   _____
26. Provided for the person's comfort.   _____ _____   _____
27. Unscreened the person.   _____ _____   _____
28. Completed a safety check before leaving the room.   _____ _____   _____
29. Practiced hand hygiene.   _____ _____   _____
30. Recorded the right documentation on the MAR:
    A. The date, time, drug name, dosage, and route of administration   _____ _____   _____
    B. Your name or initials   _____ _____   _____
31. Reported and recorded any specific patient or resident observations or concerns.   _____ _____   _____

Date of Satisfactory Completion _____   Instructor's Initials _____

Giving an Oral Drug—Liquid Form

Name: _____		Date: _____

Quality of Life	S	U	Comments

Remembered to:
- Knock before entering the person's room.
- Address the person by name.
- Introduce yourself by name and title.
- Explain the procedure to the person before beginning and during the procedure.
- Protect the person's rights during the procedure.
- Handle the person gently during the procedure.

Pre-Procedure

1. Checked the drug order. (First safety check.) Focused on the right drug, right time, right dose, right person, right route.
2. Checked with the nurse if you had any questions.
3. Practiced hand hygiene.
4. Collected the following:
   A. MAR
   B. Medicine cup
   C. Oral syringe, if needed, in the correct size
   D. Tray, if needed
   E. Paper towels
5. Unlocked the drug cart.
6. Read the order on the MAR.
7. Selected the right drug from the person's drawer or bin.
8. Compared the drug order on the MAR against the pharmacy label on the drug container. (Second safety check.) Checked for the right drug, right time, right dose, right person, right route.
9. Checked the drug container for an expiration date.
10. Compared the drug order on the MAR against the pharmacy label on the drug container. (Third safety check.) Checked for the right drug, right time, right dose, right person, right route.
11. Prepared the drug: (Did not open a unit dose container until at the bedside.)
    A. Shook the bottle or container only if directed to do so on the label.
    B. Opened the container. Did not open a unit dose container until at the person's bedside.
    C. Placed the lid on the drug cart. The outside of lid was down; the inside of the lid was up.
    D. Held the bottle so the label was is in the palm of your hand.
12. For a *medicine cup:*
    A. Located the scale to be used on the medicine cup.
    B. Placed your fingernail at the level to be measured.
    C. Held the medicine cup straight at eye level.
    D. Poured the prescribed dose into the medicine cup.
    E. Compared the drug order on the MAR against the pharmacy label on the drug container.
    F. Set the medicine cup on the drug cart.

Date of Satisfactory Completion _____		Instructor's Initials _____

Procedure—cont'd	S	U	Comments
13. For a *syringe*:			
A. Followed steps 12 A-F.	___	___	_____
B. Pulled back on the plunger to withdraw the drug from the medicine cup into the barrel.	___	___	_____
C. Set the syringe on the tray or a paper towel.	___	___	_____
14. Wiped off any liquid from the bottle top.	___	___	_____
15. Replaced the lid on the bottle.	___	___	_____
16. Closed the bottle. Compared the drug order on the MAR against the pharmacy label on the drug container. (Fourth safety check.) Checked for the right drug, right time, right dose, right person, right route.	___	___	_____
17. Returned the bottle to the drawer or bin.	___	___	_____
18. Repeated steps 6-17 for each liquid drug ordered for the person.	___	___	_____
19. Locked the drug cart if left outside the person's room.	___	___	_____

Procedure

	S	U	Comments
20. Identified the person. Checked the ID bracelet against the MAR. Used at least two identifiers according to agency policy. Called the person by name. Followed agency policy if bar code scanner used.	___	___	_____
21. Provided for privacy.	___	___	_____
22. Obtained required measurements as noted on the MAR. Noted the measurement on the MAR.	___	___	_____
23. Positioned the person in a sitting or Fowler's position. Or positioned the person as directed by the nurse, care plan, and MAR.	___	___	_____
24. Gave the person the medicine cup.	___	___	_____
25. For a *unit dose system*:			
A. Handed the drug container to the person. Asked him or her to read the label.	___	___	_____
B. Asked the person to hand the container back to you.	___	___	_____
C. Opened the container.	___	___	_____
D Gave the container to the person.	___	___	_____
E. Have the person drink the drug.	___	___	_____
26. For a *medicine dropper or an oral syringe*:			
A. Placed the dropper or syringe inside the mouth by the tongue.	___	___	_____
B Gave the liquid in small amounts. Allowed time for the person to swallow.	___	___	_____
C Returned the dropper to the bottle.	___	___	_____

Post-Procedure

	S	U	Comments
25. Discarded the medicine cup, unit dose container, or oral syringe.	___	___	_____
26. Provided for the person's comfort.	___	___	_____
27. Unscreened the person.	___	___	_____
28. Completed a safety check before leaving the room.	___	___	_____
29. Practiced hand hygiene.	___	___	_____
30. Recorded the right documentation on the MAR:			
A. The date, time, drug name, dosage, and route of administration	___	___	_____
B. Your name or initials	___	___	_____
31. Reported and recorded any specific patient or resident observations or concerns	___	___	_____

Date of Satisfactory Completion _____   Instructor's Initials _____

Applying a Cream, Lotion, Ointment, or Powder

Name: _____   Date: _____

Quality of Life	S	U	Comments
Remembered to:			
• Knock before entering the person's room.			
• Address the person by name.			
• Introduce yourself by name and title.			
• Explain the procedure to the person before beginning and during the procedure.			
• Protect the person's rights during the procedure.			
• Handle the person gently during the procedure.			

Pre-Procedure

	S	U	Comments
1. Followed *Delegation Guidelines: Applying Creams, Lotions, Ointments, and Powders.* Viewed *Promoting Safety and Comfort: Applying Creams, Lotions, Ointments, and Powders.*			
2. Checked the drug order. (First safety check.) Focused on the right drug, right time, right dose, right person, right route.			
3. Checked with the nurse if you had any questions.			
4. Practiced hand hygiene.			
5. Collected needed items:			
A. Soap or other cleansing agent			
B. Washcloth and towel			
C. Wash basin with warm water			
D. Gauze square or cotton balls			
E. Sterile tongue blade			
F. Sterile cotton-tipped applicator			
G. Gloves			
H. MAR			

Procedure

	S	U	Comments
6. Unlocked the drug cart.			
7. Read the order on the MAR.			
8. Selected the right drug from the person's drawer. Locked the drug cart.			
9. Compared the drug order on the MAR against the pharmacy label on the drug container. (Second safety check.) Checked for the right drug, right time, right dose, right person, right route.			
10. Checked the drug container for an expiration date.			
11. Identified the person. Checked the ID bracelet against the MAR. Used at least two identifiers according to agency policy. Called the person by name. Followed agency policy if bar code scanner used.			
12. Provided for privacy.			
13. Put on gloves.			
14. Positioned the person to expose the application site. Exposed the site.			
15. Cleaned and dried the application site.			
16. Observed the application site.			
17. Removed and discarded the gloves. Practiced hand hygiene. Put on clean gloves.			
18. Compared the drug order on the MAR against the pharmacy label on the drug container. (Third safety check.) Checked for the right drug, right time, right dose, right person, right route.			

Date of Satisfactory Completion _____   Instructor's Initials _____

Procedure—cont'd	S	U	Comments

19. Shook lotion thoroughly.
20. Opened the container. Placed the lid or cap upside down on a clean surface. For an *ointment or cream*:
    A. From a jar: used a tongue blade to remove the ordered amount.
    B. From a tube: squeezed the ordered amount onto a tongue blade or cotton-tipped applicator.
21. Closed the container. Compared the drug order on the MAR against the pharmacy label on the drug container. (Fourth safety check.) Checked for the right drug, right time, right dose, right person, right route.
22. Applied the *lotion*:
    A. Held the bottle in your non-dominant hand with the label in your palm.
    B. Poured some lotion onto a cotton ball or gauze square. Did not let any part of the container touch the cotton ball.
    C. Dabbed the lotion onto the skin. Did not rub.
    D. Repeated steps 22 A-C with a new cotton ball or gauze square until the area was covered.
23. Applied *cream or ointment*:
    A. Transferred the cream or ointment from the tongue blade or cotton-tipped applicator to your gloved index finger.
    B. Applied the agent to the skin with your gloved finger.
    C. Applied the agent in a thin layer in the direction of hair growth. Used firm, gentle strokes.
24. Applied *powder*:
    A. Applied in a thin, even layer with your gloved hand.
    B. Smoothed over the area for even coverage.
25. Returned the container to the drawer. Locked the drug cart.

Post-Procedure
26. Discarded the supplies or unit dose packages.
27. Removed the gloves. Practiced hand hygiene.
28. Provided for the person's comfort.
29. Emptied and cleaned the wash basin. Returned it and other supplies to their proper place. Wore gloves.
30. Unscreened the person.
31. Completed a safety check before leaving the room.
32. Followed agency policy for soiled linen.
33. Practiced hand hygiene.
34. Recorded the right documentation on the MAR:
    A. The date, time, drug name, dosage, and route of administration.
    B. The application site.
    C. Your name or initials.
35. Reported and recorded any specific patient or resident observations or concerns.

Date of Satisfactory Completion _____   Instructor's Initials _____

Applying Nitroglycerine Ointment

Name: _____   Date: _____

Quality of Life	S	U	Comments

Remembered to:
- Knock before entering the person's room.
- Address the person by name.
- Introduce yourself by name and title.
- Explain the procedure to the person before beginning and during the procedure.
- Protect the person's rights during the procedure.
- Handle the person gently during the procedure.

Pre-Procedure

1. Followed *Delegation Guidelines: Applying Creams, Lotions, Ointments, and Powders.* Viewed *Promoting Safety and Comfort:*
   A. *Applying Creams, Lotions, Ointments, and Powders*
   B. *Applying Nitroglycerin Ointment*
2. Checked the drug order. (First safety check.) Focused on the right drug, right time, right dose, right person, right route.
3. Checked with the nurse if you had any questions.
4. Practiced hand hygiene.
5. Collected needed items:
   A. Soap or other cleansing agent
   B. Washcloth and towel
   C. Wash basin with warm water
   D. Applicator paper
   E. See-through dressing
   F. Non-allergic tape
   G. Gloves
   H. MAR

Procedure

6. Unlocked the drug cart.
7. Read the order on the MAR.
8. Selected the nitroglycerin ointment from the person's drawer. Locked the drug cart.
9. Compared the drug order on the MAR against the pharmacy label on the drug container. (Second safety check.) Checked for the right drug, right time, right dose, right person, right route.
10. Checked the drug container for an expiration date.
11. Provided for privacy.
12. Identified the person. Checked the ID bracelet against the MAR. Used at least two identifiers according to agency policy. Called the person by name. Followed agency policy if bar code scanner used.
13. Put on gloves.
14. Positioned the person to expose the old application site. Exposed the site.
15. Removed the old application. Folded the old application in half with the sticky sides together. Discarded the application according to agency policy. Made sure that no one could access the old application.
16. Cleaned and dried the old application site.
17. Observed the old application site.

Date of Satisfactory Completion _____   Instructor's Initials _____

Procedure—cont'd	S	U	Comments
18. Positioned the person to expose the new application site. Exposed and observed the site.	___	___	_____
19. Cleaned and dried the new application site. Followed agency policy.	___	___	_____
20. Removed and discarded the gloves. Practiced hand hygiene.	___	___	_____
21. Put on clean gloves.	___	___	_____
22. Compared the drug order on the MAR against the pharmacy label on the drug container. (Third safety check.) Checked for the right drug, right time, right dose, right person, right route.	___	___	_____
23. Used the dose-measuring paper to measure the ordered dose. Placed the print side down.	___	___	_____
24. Squeezed a ribbon of ointment on the paper for the amount ordered.	___	___	_____
25. Closed the container. Compared the drug order on the MAR against the pharmacy label on the drug container. (Fourth safety check.) Checked for the right drug, right time, right dose, right person, right route.	___	___	_____
26. Applied the paper, ointment side down, to the application site.	___	___	_____
27. Used the paper to spread a thin, uniform layer of ointment under the paper. Did not rub in the ointment.	___	___	_____
28. Left the paper in place.	___	___	_____
29. Covered the paper and application site with a see-through dressing. Taped the dressing in place.	___	___	_____
30. Dated, timed, and signed your name and title to the tape. Include the drug name and dosage.	___	___	_____
31. Returned the container to the drawer. Locked the drug cart.	___	___	_____

Post-Procedure

	S	U	Comments
32. Discarded the supplies.	___	___	_____
33. Removed the gloves. Practiced hand hygiene.	___	___	_____
34. Provided for the person's comfort.	___	___	_____
35. Emptied and cleaned the wash basin. Returned it and other supplies to their proper place. Wore gloves.	___	___	_____
36. Unscreened the person.	___	___	_____
37. Completed a safety check before leaving the room.	___	___	_____
38. Followed agency policy for soiled linen.	___	___	_____
39. Practiced hand hygiene.	___	___	_____
40. Recorded the right documentation on the MAR:			
A. The removal of an old application and from what site.	___	___	_____
B. The date, time, drug name, dosage, and route of administration	___	___	_____
C. The application site	___	___	_____
D. Your name or initials	___	___	_____
41. Reported and recorded any specific patient or resident observations or concerns.	___	___	_____

Date of Satisfactory Completion _____   Instructor's Initials _____

Applying Medications to the Eye

Name: _____   Date: _____

Quality of Life	S	U	Comments

Remembered to:
- Knock before entering the person's room.
- Address the person by name.
- Introduce yourself by name and title.
- Explain the procedure to the person before beginning and during the procedure.
- Protect the person's rights during the procedure.
- Handle the person gently during the procedure.

Pre-Procedure
1. Followed *Delegation Guidelines: Eye Medications.* Viewed *Promoting Safety and Comfort: Eye Medications.*
2. Checked the drug order. (First safety check.) Focused on the right drug, right time, right dose, right person, right route.
3. Checked with the nurse if you had any questions.
4. Practiced hand hygiene.
5. Collected needed items:
   A. Gauze squares, cotton balls, or a washcloth
   B. Saline solution
   C. Tissues
   D. Gloves
   E. MAR

Procedure
6. Unlocked the drug cart.
7. Read the order on the MAR.
8. Selected the right drug from the person's drawer. Locked the drug cart.
9. Compared the drug order on the MAR against the pharmacy label on the drug container. (Second safety check.) Checked for the right drug, right time, right dose, right person, right route.
10. Checked the drug container for an expiration date.
11. Provided for privacy.
12. Identified the person. Checked the ID bracelet against the MAR. Used at least two identifiers according to agency policy. Called the person by name. Followed agency policy if bar code scanner used.
13. Put on gloves.
14. Positioned the person supine or in a sitting position. The head was tilted back slightly.
15. Removed eye drainage. Cleaned from the inner aspect to the outer aspect. Used a new gauze square or cotton ball with saline for each wipe. If a washcloth was used, a clean part of the washcloth was used for each wipe.
16. Observed the eye.
17. Compared the drug order on the MAR against the pharmacy label on the drug container. (Third safety check.) Checked for the right drug, right time, right dose, right person, right route
18. Opened the container. For ointment, placed the lid or cap upside down on a clean surface.
19. Compared the drug order on the MAR against the pharmacy label on the drug container. (Fourth safety check.) This was done before applying the dose. Checked for the right drug, right time, right dose, right person, right route.

Date of Satisfactory Completion _____   Instructor's Initials _____

Procedure—cont'd	S	U	Comments
20. Asked the person to look up toward the ceiling.	____	____	_____
21. Exposed the lower conjunctival sac with your non-dominant hand. Gently pulled down on the lower lid. Used a gauze square, cotton ball, or tissue if desired.	____	____	_____
22. Applied *eye drops*:			
A. Held the container in your dominant hand.	____	____	_____
B. Held the dropper ½ to ¾ inches above the conjunctival sac.	____	____	_____
C. Dropped the ordered number of drops into the conjunctival sac.	____	____	_____
D. Released the lid.	____	____	_____
E. Applied gentle pressure to the inner corner of the eyelid on the bone for 1 to 2 minutes. Used a clean cotton ball or tissue.	____	____	_____
23. Applied *eye ointment*:	____	____	_____
A. Squeezed the ointment in a strip fashion into the conjunctival sac. Started at the inner aspect and moved toward the outer aspect.	____	____	_____
B. Asked the person to gently close his or her eyes and move the eyes as if looking around the room.	____	____	_____
24. Capped and returned the container to the drawer. Locked the drug cart.	____	____	_____

Post-Procedure

	S	U	Comments
25. Discarded the supplies or unit dose packages.	____	____	_____
26. Removed the gloves. Practiced hand hygiene.	____	____	_____
27. Provided for the person's comfort.	____	____	_____
28. Unscreened the person.	____	____	_____
29. Completed a safety check before leaving the room.	____	____	_____
30. Followed agency policy for soiled linen.	____	____	_____
31. Practiced hand hygiene.	____	____	_____
32. Recorded the right documentation on the MAR:			
A. The date, time, drug name, dosage, and route of administration	____	____	_____
B. The application site	____	____	_____
C. Your name or initials	____	____	_____
33. Reported and recorded any specific patient or resident observations or concerns.	____	____	_____

Date of Satisfactory Completion _____   Instructor's Initials _____

Instilling Ear Drops

Name: _____   Date: _____

Quality of Life	S	U	Comments

Remembered to:
- Knock before entering the person's room.
- Address the person by name.
- Introduce yourself by name and title.
- Explain the procedure to the person before beginning and during the procedure.
- Protect the person's rights during the procedure.
- Handle the person gently during the procedure.

Pre-Procedure
1. Followed *Delegation Guidelines: Ear Medications.* Viewed *Promoting Safety and Comfort: Ear Medications.*
2. Checked the drug order. (First safety check.) Focused on the right drug, right time, right dose, right person, right route.
3. Checked with the nurse if you had any questions.
4. Practiced hand hygiene.
5. Collected needed items:
   A. Wet washcloth
   B. Cotton pledget or plug
   C. Gloves
   D. MAR

Procedure
6. Unlocked the drug cart.
7. Read the order on the MAR.
8. Selected the right drug from the person's drawer. Locked the drug cart.
9. Compared the drug order on the MAR against the pharmacy label on the drug container. (Second safety check.) Checked for the right drug, right time, right dose, right person, right route.
10. Checked the drug container for an expiration date.
11. Provided for privacy.
12. Identified the person. Checked the ID bracelet against the MAR. Used at least two identifiers according to agency policy. Called the person by name. Followed agency policy if bar code scanner used.
13. Put on gloves.
14. Positioned the person in a side-lying position. The affected ear was up.
15. Removed excess ear wax. Used the wet washcloth.
16. Observed the ear.
17. Compared the drug order on the MAR against the pharmacy label on the drug container. (Third safety check.) Checked for the right drug, right time, right dose, right person, right route.
18. Opened the container.
19. Drew medication into the dropper.
20. Compared the drug order on the MAR against the pharmacy label on the drug container. (Fourth safety check.) Checked for the right drug, right time, right dose, right person, right route.

Date of Satisfactory Completion _____   Instructor's Initials _____

Procedure—cont'd	S	U	Comments
21. Applied ear drops (for persons 3 years of age and older):			
A. Pulled the ear upward and back.	___	___	_____
B. Instilled the ordered number of drops along the side of the ear canal.	___	___	_____
C. Returned the dropper to the container.	___	___	_____
22. Inserted a cotton pledget or plug loosely into the ear if ordered.	___	___	_____
23. Asked the person to remain in the side-lying position for 5 to 10 minutes, or as directed by the nurse and care plan.	___	___	_____
24. Removed the cotton pledget or plug.	___	___	_____
25. Returned the container to the drawer. Locked the drug cart.	___	___	_____

Post-Procedure

	S	U	Comments
26. Discarded the supplies or unit dose packages.	___	___	_____
27. Removed the gloves. Practiced hand hygiene.	___	___	_____
28. Provided for the person's comfort.	___	___	_____
29. Unscreened the person.	___	___	_____
30. Completed a safety check before leaving the room.	___	___	_____
31. Followed agency policy for soiled linen.	___	___	_____
32. Practiced hand hygiene.	___	___	_____
33. Recorded the right documentation on the MAR:			
A. The date, time, drug name, dosage, and route of administration	___	___	_____
B. The application site	___	___	_____
C. Your name or initials	___	___	_____
34. Reported and recorded any specific patient or resident observations or concerns.	___	___	_____

Date of Satisfactory Completion _____ Instructor's Initials _____

Giving Nose Medications

Name: _____

Date: _____

Quality of Life	S	U	Comments

Remembered to:
- Knock before entering the person's room.
- Address the person by name.
- Introduce yourself by name and title.
- Explain the procedure to the person before beginning and during the procedure.
- Protect the person's rights during the procedure.
- Handle the person gently during the procedure.

Pre-Procedure
1. Followed *Delegation Guidelines: Nose Medications.* Viewed *Promoting Safety and Comfort: Nose Medications.*
2. Checked the drug order. (First safety check.) Focused on the right drug, right time, right dose, right person, right route.
3. Checked with the nurse if you had any questions.
4. Practiced hand hygiene.
5. Collected needed items:
    A. Tissues
    B. Gloves
    C. MAR

Procedure
6. Unlocked the drug cart.
7. Read the order on the MAR.
8. Selected the right drug from the person's drawer. Locked the drug cart.
9. Compared the drug order on the MAR against the pharmacy label on the drug container. (Second safety check.) Checked for the right drug, right time, right dose, right person, right route.
10. Checked the drug container for an expiration date.
11. Provided for privacy.
12. Identified the person. Checked the ID bracelet against the MAR. Used at least two identifiers according to agency policy. Called the person by name. Followed agency policy if bar code scanner used.
13. Put on gloves.
14. Observed the nose.
15. Compared the drug order on the MAR against the pharmacy label on the drug container. (Third safety check.) Checked for the right drug, right time, right dose, right person, right route.
16. Opened the container. For nasal spray, placed the lid or cap upside down on a clean surface.
17. Compared the drug order on the MAR against the pharmacy label on the drug container. (Fourth safety check.) This was done before applying the dose. Checked for the right drug, right time, right dose, right person, right route.

Date of Satisfactory Completion _____   Instructor's Initials _____

Procedure—cont'd	S	U	Comments
18. Gave *nose drops (for adults and older children)*:			
A. Asked the person to gently blow the nose. Provided tissues.	___ ___		_____
B. Positioned the person supine with the head over the edge of the mattress. Or positioned the person as directed by the nurse and the care plan.	___ ___		_____
C. Drew medication into the dropper.	___ ___		_____
D. Held the dropper about ½ inch above the nostril.	___ ___		_____
E. Instilled the number of drops ordered.	___ ___		_____
F. Repeated steps 18 A-E for the other nostril.	___ ___		_____
G. Asked the person to remain as positioned for 5 minutes or for as long as directed by the nurse and the care plan.	___ ___		_____
19. Gave *nasal spray*:			
A. Asked the person to gently blow the nose. Provided tissues.	___ ___		_____
B. Positioned the person in a sitting or Fowler's position.	___ ___		_____
C. Blocked one nostril.	___ ___		_____
D. Held the spray bottle upright. Shook the bottle.	___ ___		_____
E. Inserted the bottle tip into the nostril.	___ ___		_____
F. Asked the person to take a deep breath.	___ ___		_____
G. Squeezed a puff of spray into the nostril as the person took a deep breath.	___ ___		_____
H. Wiped the bottle tip before spraying the other nostril. Then repeated steps 19 A-G.	___ ___		_____
20. Provided the person with tissues for blotting drainage. Reminded the person not to blow his or her nose for several minutes.	___ ___		_____
21. Returned the container to the drawer. Locked the drug cart.	___ ___		_____
Post-Procedure			
22. Discarded the supplies or unit dose packages.	___ ___		_____
23. Removed the gloves. Practiced hand hygiene.	___ ___		_____
24. Provided for the person's comfort.	___ ___		_____
25. Unscreened the person.	___ ___		_____
26. Completed a safety check before leaving the room.	___ ___		_____
27. Followed agency policy for soiled linen.	___ ___		_____
28. Practiced hand hygiene.	___ ___		_____
29. Recorded the right documentation on the MAR:			
A. The date, time, drug name, dosage, and route of administration	___ ___		_____
B. The application site	___ ___		_____
C. Your name or initials	___ ___		_____
30. Reported and recorded any specific patient or resident observations or concerns.	___ ___		_____

Date of Satisfactory Completion _____   Instructor's Initials _____

Giving Inhaled Medications

Name: _____   Date: _____

Quality of Life	S	U	Comments

Remembered to:
- Knock before entering the person's room.
- Address the person by name.
- Introduce yourself by name and title.
- Explain the procedure to the person before beginning and during the procedure.
- Protect the person's rights during the procedure.
- Handle the person gently during the procedure.

Pre-Procedure
1. Followed *Delegation Guidelines: Inhaled Medications.* Viewed *Promoting Safety and Comfort: Inhaled Medications.*
2. Checked the drug order. (First safety check.) Focused on the right drug, right time, right dose, right person, right route.
3. Checked with the nurse if you had any questions.
4. Practiced hand hygiene.
5. Collected needed items:
   A. Tissues
   B. Gloves
   C. MAR

Procedure
6. Unlocked the drug cart.
7. Read the order on the MAR.
8. Selected the right inhaler from the person's drawer. Locked the drug cart.
9. Compared the drug order on the MAR against the pharmacy label on the inhaler. (Second safety check.) Checked for the right drug, right time, right dose, right person, right route.
10. Checked the inhaler for an expiration date.
11. Provided for privacy.
12. Identified the person. Checked the ID bracelet against the MAR. Used at least two identifiers according to agency policy. Called the person by name. Followed agency policy if bar code scanner used.
13. Put on gloves.
14. Compared the drug order on the MAR against the pharmacy label on the inhaler. (Third safety check.) Checked for the right drug, right time, right dose, right person, right route.
15. Positioned the person so that he or she is upright—standing, sitting, or Fowler's position.
16. Removed the cap from the inhaler. Placed the lid or cap upside down on a clean surface.
17. Compared the drug order on the MAR against the pharmacy label on the inhaler. (Fourth safety check.) Checked for the right drug, right time, right dose, right person, right route.
18. Held the inhaler upright. Used thumb and first one or two fingers to give the drug.

Date of Satisfactory Completion _____   Instructor's Initials _____

Procedure—cont'd	S	U	Comments
19. Gave *MDI without a spacer:*			
A. Shook the inhaler the number of times as directed by the nurse.	_____	_____	_____
B. Asked the person to open his or her mouth. Asked the person to tilt his or her head back slightly.	_____	_____	_____
C. Asked the person to exhale.	_____	_____	_____
D. Placed the inhaler 1 to 2 inches in front of the person's mouth.	_____	_____	_____
E. Pushed down on or squeezed the dispensing valve. Asked the person to inhale deeply and slowly for 3 to 5 seconds.	_____	_____	_____
F. Asked the person to hold his or her breath for about 10 seconds.	_____	_____	_____
G. Asked the person to exhale slowly through his or her mouth.	_____	_____	_____
H. Repeated the puffs as ordered. Shook the inhaler again. Repeated steps 19 A-G.	_____	_____	_____
20. Gave *MDI with a spacer:*			
A. Inserted the inhaler into the spacer.	_____	_____	_____
B. Shook the inhaler and spacer the number of times as directed by the nurse.	_____	_____	_____
C. Asked the person to open his or her mouth. Asked the person to tilt his or her head back slightly.	_____	_____	_____
D. Asked the person to exhale.	_____	_____	_____
E. Asked the person to place the spacer mouthpiece in his her mouth. Then asked the person to close the lips around the mouthpiece.	_____	_____	_____
F. Pushed down on or squeezed the dispensing valve. Asked the person to inhale deeply and slowly for 3 to 5 seconds.	_____	_____	_____
G. Asked the person to hold his or her breath for about 10 seconds.	_____	_____	_____
H. Asked the person to exhale slowly through his or her mouth.	_____	_____	_____
I. Repeated the puffs as ordered. Shook the inhaler again. Repeat steps 20 A-H.	_____	_____	_____
21. Removed the spacer (if used). Replaced the cap on the inhaler.	_____	_____	_____
22. Had the person rinse his or her mouth with water if he or she inhaled a cortico-steroid.	_____	_____	_____
23. Returned the inhaler and spacer to the drawer. Locked the drug cart.	_____	_____	_____

Post-Procedure

	S	U	Comments
24. Removed the gloves. Practiced hand hygiene.	_____	_____	_____
25. Provided for the person's comfort.	_____	_____	_____
26. Unscreened the person.	_____	_____	_____
27. Cleaned the inhaler and spacer. Followed the manufacturer's instructions. Wore gloves.	_____	_____	_____
28. Completed a safety check before leaving the room.	_____	_____	_____
29. Followed agency policy for soiled linen.	_____	_____	_____
30. Practiced hand hygiene.	_____	_____	_____
31. Recorded the right documentation on the MAR:			
A. The date, time, drug name, dosage, and route of administration	_____	_____	_____
B. The application site	_____	_____	_____
C. Your name or initials	_____	_____	_____
32. Reported and recorded any specific patient or resident observations or concerns.	_____	_____	_____

Date of Satisfactory Completion _____   Instructor's Initials _____

Giving Vaginal Drugs

Name: _____   Date: _____

Quality of Life	S	U	Comments

Remembered to:
- Knock before entering the person's room.
- Address the person by name.
- Introduce yourself by name and title.
- Explain the procedure to the person before beginning and during the procedure.
- Protect the person's rights during the procedure.
- Handle the person gently during the procedure.

Pre-Procedure
1. Followed *Delegation Guidelines: Vaginal Drugs.* Viewed *Promoting Safety and Comfort: Vaginal Drugs.*
2. Checked the drug order. (First safety check.) Focused on the right drug, right time, right dose, right person, right route.
3. Checked with the nurse if you had any questions.
4. Practiced hand hygiene.
5. Collected needed items:
   - A. Vaginal applicator
   - B. Water-soluble lubricant
   - C. Pillow
   - D. Perineal pad or panty shield
   - E. Gloves
   - F. Paper towels
   - G. MAR

Procedure
6. Unlocked the drug cart or storage area.
7. Read the order on the MAR.
8. Selected the right drug from the person's drawer or the storage area. Locked the drug cart or storage area.
9. Compared the drug order on the MAR against the pharmacy label on the drug container. (Second safety check.) Checked for the right drug, right time, right dose, right person, right route.
10. Checked the drug container for an expiration date.
11. Provided for privacy.
12. Identified the person. Checked the ID bracelet against the MAR. Used at least two identifiers according to agency policy. Called the person by name. Followed agency policy if bar code scanner used.
13. Put on gloves.
14. Positioned and draped the woman in the lithotomy position. Elevated her hips on a pillow.
15. Removed and discarded the gloves. Practiced hand hygiene. Put on clean gloves.
16. Compared the drug order on the MAR against the pharmacy label on the drug container. (Third safety check.) Checked for the right drug, right time, right dose, right person, right route.

Date of Satisfactory Completion _____   Instructor's Initials _____

	S	U	Comments

Procedure—cont'd

17. Prepared the drug—*cream, foam, or gel with an applicator:*
    A. Opened the container. Placed the lid or cap upside down on a clean surface.
    B. Attached the applicator to the container.
    C. Squeezed the container to fill the applicator.
    D. Lubricated the applicator tip. Used water-soluble lubricant.
    E. Set the applicator on a paper towel.
18. Prepared the drug—*suppository:*
    A. Opened and removed the wrapper containing the suppository.
    B. Inserted the suppository into an applicator (if using one).
    C. Lubricated the suppository. Used water-soluble lubricant.
    D. Set the suppository on a paper towel.
19. Closed the container. Compared the drug order on the MAR against the pharmacy label on the drug container. (Fourth safety check.) Checked for the right drug, right time, right dose, right person, right route.
20. Exposed the perineum.
21. Observed the perineum and vaginal opening.
22. Administered the dose form—*cream, foam, or gel with an applicator:*
    A. Spread the labia to expose the vagina. Used non-dominant hand.
    B. Inserted the applicator as far as possible into the vagina.
    C. Pushed the plunger to deposit the drug.
    D. Removed the applicator.
    E. Wrapped the applicator in the paper towel.
23. Administered the dose form—*suppository:*
    A. Lubricated your gloved index finger (if not using an applicator). Used water-soluble lubricant.
    B. Spread the labia to expose the vagina. Used non-dominant hand.
    C. Inserted the suppository as far as possible into the vagina. Used gloved finger or an applicator.
    D. Removed the applicator (if used).
    E. Wrapped the applicator (if used) in the paper towel.
24. Applied a perineal pad or panty shield.
25. Assisted the woman to the supine position with her hips elevated. Asked her to remain in this position for 5 to 10 minutes, or as directed by the nurse, care plan, or MAR.
26. Removed and discarded the gloves.
27. Practiced hand hygiene.
28. Returned the container to the drawer or storage area. Locked the drug cart or storage area.

Post-Procedure

29. Discarded supplies or unit dose packages.
30. Provided for the person's comfort.
31. Unscreened the person.
32. Emptied and cleaned the applicator. Stored it according to agency policy. Discarded the paper towel. Wore gloves.
33. Completed a safety check before leaving the room.
34. Followed agency policy for soiled linen.
35. Practiced hand hygiene.
36. Recorded the right documentation on the MAR:
    A. The date, time, drug name, dosage, and route of administration
    B. The application site
    C. Your name or initials
37. Reported and recorded any specific patient or resident observations or concerns.

Date of Satisfactory Completion _____   Instructor's Initials _____

Giving a Rectal Suppository

Name: _____   Date: _____

Quality of Life	S	U	Comments

Remembered to:
- Knock before entering the person's room.
- Address the person by name.
- Introduce yourself by name and title.
- Explain the procedure to the person before beginning and during the procedure.
- Protect the person's rights during the procedure.
- Handle the person gently during the procedure.

Pre-Procedure
1. Followed *Delegation Guidelines: Rectal Drugs.* Viewed *Promoting Safety and Comfort: Rectal Drugs.*
2. Checked the drug order. (First safety check.) Focused on the right drug, right time, right dose, right person, right route.
3. Checked with the nurse if you had any questions.
4. Practiced hand hygiene.
5. Collected needed items:
   A. Water-soluble lubricant
   B. Gloves
   C. Paper towels
   D. Toilet tissue
   E. MAR

Procedure
6. Unlocked the drug cart or the storage area.
7. Read the order on the MAR.
8. Selected the right drug from the storage area. Locked the storage area.
9. Compared the drug order on the MAR against the pharmacy label on the drug container. (Second safety check.) Checked for the right drug, right time, right dose, right person, right route.
10. Checked the drug container for an expiration date.
11. Provided for privacy.
12. Identified the person. Checked the ID bracelet against the MAR. Used at least two identifiers according to agency policy. Called the person by name. Followed agency policy if bar code scanner used.
13. Put on gloves.
14. Positioned and draped the person in Sims' position or a left side-lying position. Bent the uppermost leg toward the waist.
15. Compared the drug order on the MAR against the pharmacy label on the drug container. (Third safety check.) Checked for the right drug, right time, right dose, right person, right route.
16. Opened and removed the wrapper containing the suppository.
17. Lubricated the suppository.
18. Set the suppository on a paper towel.

Date of Satisfactory Completion _____   Instructor's Initials _____

	S	U	Comments
Procedure—cont'd			
19. Compared the drug order on the MAR against the pharmacy label on the drug container. (Fourth safety check.) Checked for the right drug, right time, right dose, right person, right route.	____	____	_____
20. Exposed the rectal area.	____	____	_____
21. Observed the rectal area.	____	____	_____
22. Inserted the suppository:			
A. Raised the upper buttock to expose the anus.	____	____	_____
B. Asked the person take a deep breath.	____	____	_____
C. Placed the rounded tip of the suppository into the anus and rectum. Inserted it about 1 inch into the rectum along the rectal wall.	____	____	_____
23. Wiped the anus to remove excess lubricant.	____	____	_____
24. Asked the person to remain in a left side-lying position for 15 to 20 minutes, or as directed by the nurse, care plan, or MAR.			
Post-Procedure			
25. Discarded supplies or unit dose packages. Disposed of toilet tissue.	____	____	_____
26. Removed and discarded the gloves. Practiced hand hygiene.	____	____	_____
27. Provided for the person's comfort.	____	____	_____
28. Unscreened the person.	____	____	_____
29. Completed a safety check before leaving the room.	____	____	_____
30. Followed agency policy for soiled linen.	____	____	_____
31. Practiced hand hygiene.	____	____	_____
32. Recorded the right documentation on the MAR:			
A. The date, time, drug name, dosage, and route of administration	____	____	_____
B. The application site	____	____	_____
C. Your name or initials	____	____	_____
33. Reported and recorded any specific patient or resident observations or concerns	____	____	_____

Date of Satisfactory Completion _____   Instructor's Initials _____

Printed in the United States
By Bookmasters